一串珍珠

STRING OF PEARLS

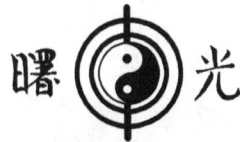

曙 ☯ 光

Twin Cities T'ai Chi Ch'uan
10th Anniversary Collection

Compiled and Edited by Ray Hayward

Ray Hayward Enterprises, LLC

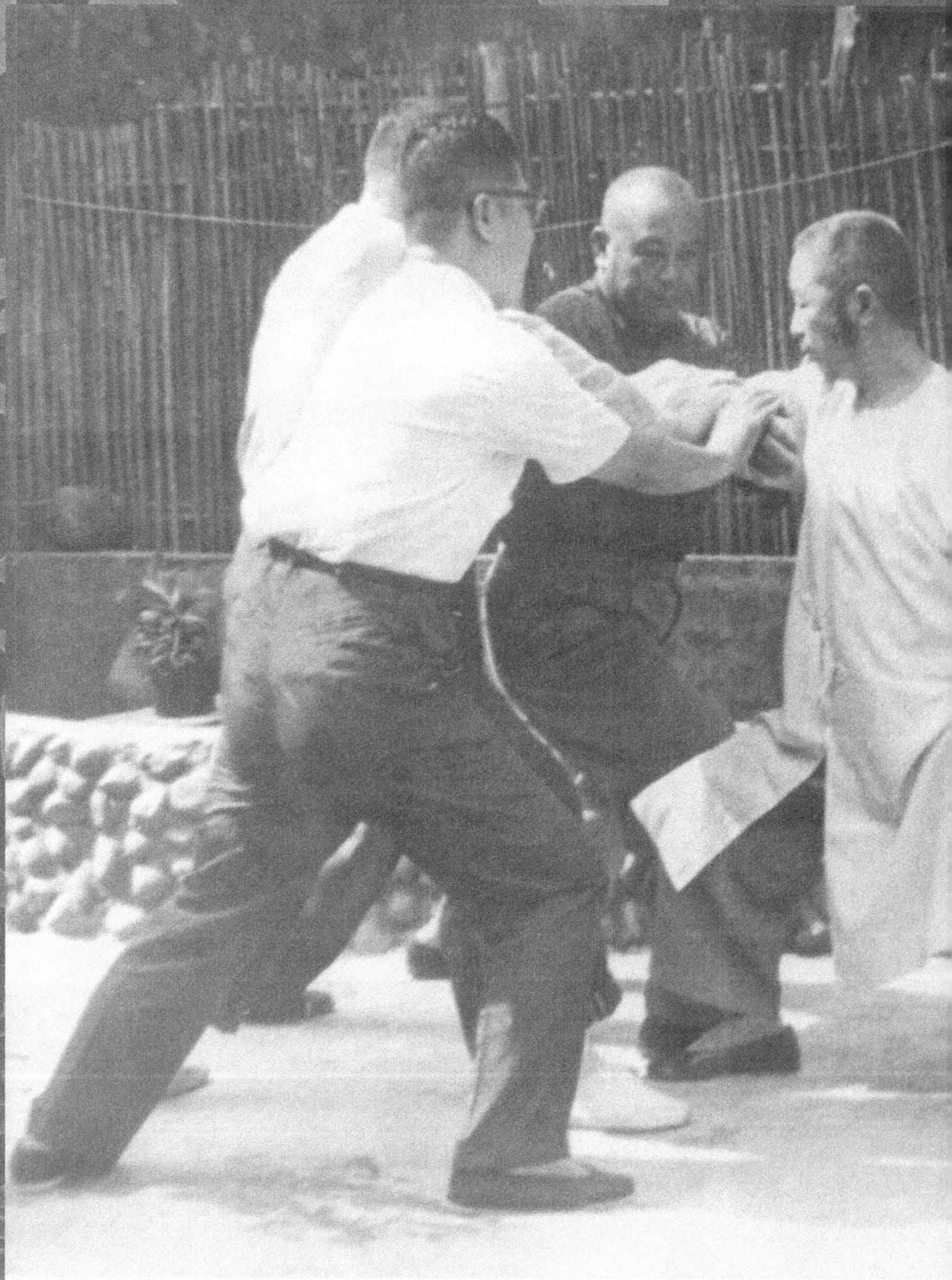

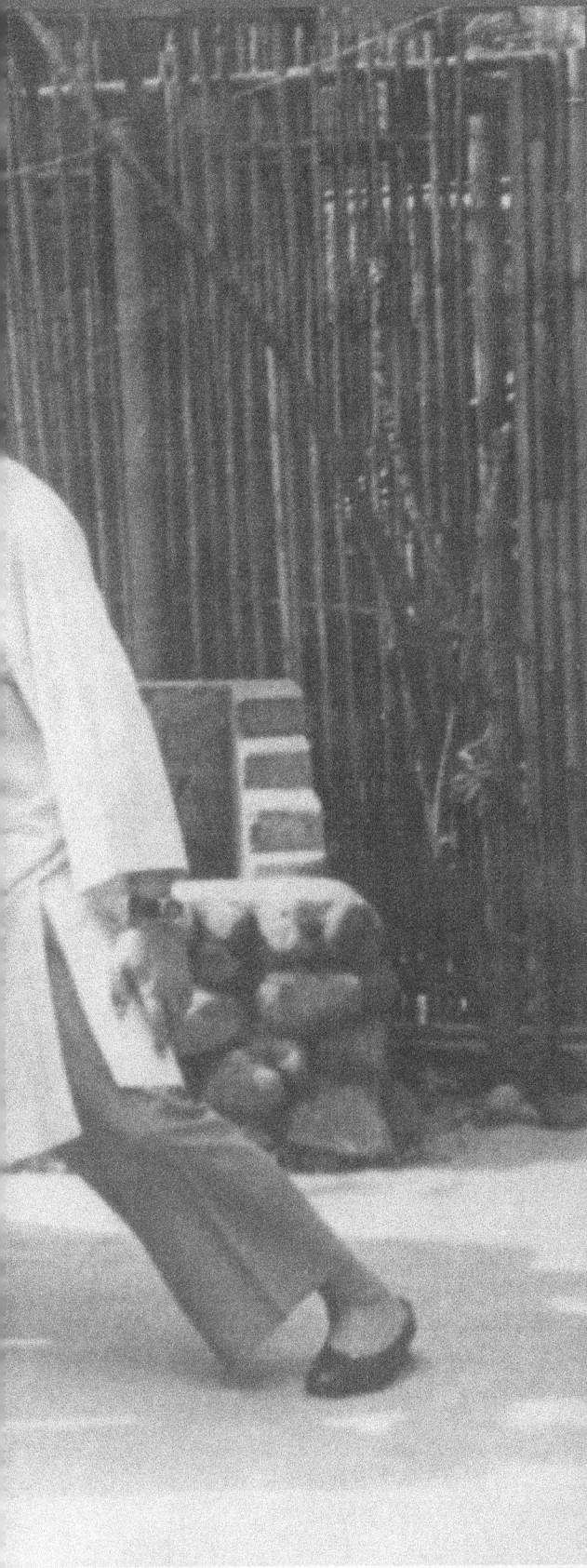

This book is dedicated to the students who came through the door looking for T'ai Chi, and found themselves.

Left: Master Cheng Man-ching roots the push of four people.

STRING OF PEARLS

First Printing – 2003.

Photographs courtesy of Master T.T. Liang, Ray Hayward, Paul Abdella, An-le Liang, Dan Polsfuss, J.R. Roy and Elyse Duffy.

Published by: **Ray Hayward Enterprises, LLC**

Disclaimer: The author and publisher of this book are not responsible for any injury that may result from following the instructions contained herein. The reader should consult his or her physician for advice before attempting any such activities.

ISBN 978-0-692-07085-7
3 4 5 6 7 8 / 23 22 21 20 19 18

Contents

INTRODUCTION

WHY YOU SHOULD STUDY T'AI-CHI

Joanne Von Blon; 7th generation lineage holder and founding Board of Directors memeber of Twin Cities T'ai Chi Ch'uan, and Studio patron, 2002

"Ray," I said, "what should I write for the anniversary?" He said, "Why don't you write what you would tell people who ask why they should take T'ai-Chi?" After 20 years of practice and at age 78, I can do that.

If they were young I would tell them that T'ai-Chi will improve their performance in any other sport they ever undertake. To be relaxed is to be fast and to be relaxed saves energy. I would tell them that T'ai-Chi is a magnificent fighting art and superb self-defense, but it takes a lot of training and they are lucky to start young.

I would add that the meditation practice would improve their concentration and lessen test anxieties. Finally, I would say that their friends would be curious and admire them for doing something a little different.

If they were closer to my age I would tell them that T'ai-Chi promises eternal Springtime, that we will carry good health into advanced old age. T'ai-Chi is moderate, safe exercise that engages every muscle group and works the mind and body as one entity. Because T'ai-Chi breathing trains the body to use oxygen more efficiently, the exercise is also aerobic. T'ai-Chi reduces stress, and stress is bad for our hearts.

Our balance will improve, lessening the likelihood of a fall. And if we should fall, our center of gravity has sunk and our relaxation response will make injury less likely. T'ai-Chi is a weight-bearing exercise that strengthens bones, lessening the danger of osteoporosis and a broken hip.

An added plus for Minnesota winters: the relaxation allows the blood to circulate through all the capillaries, keeping our hands and feet warmer. When we learn "reverse breathing" we warm up even faster.

For the majority of students in the middle age ranges, all of the above holds true and T'ai-Chi holds even more satisfactions. First, there is the discipline and fun of learning the Solo Form, something entirely new. This is followed, as we learn to relax, by the satisfaction of measurable progress. These epiphanies may be the best part of T'ai-Chi and they continue to happen from time to time for as long as we practice.

Those of us who go on to further study can learn sword, spear, cane and other weapons; we practice "pushing hands;" we learn the "two-person dance." Many of us begin to tutor other students, which adds to our own knowledge and pleasure. We meet the challenges of overcoming inevitable plateaus, and most importantly, the real joy and excitement of sudden insights, the knowledge that suddenly you did it right!

If any persons were still listening, I'd tell them two more things. One, that I treasure doing T'ai-Chi with and knowing an astounding diversity of men and women. And finally, I would say that in all their lives they will seldom meet a finer man, a better martial artist, or a funnier, more imaginative, or more creative teacher than mine.

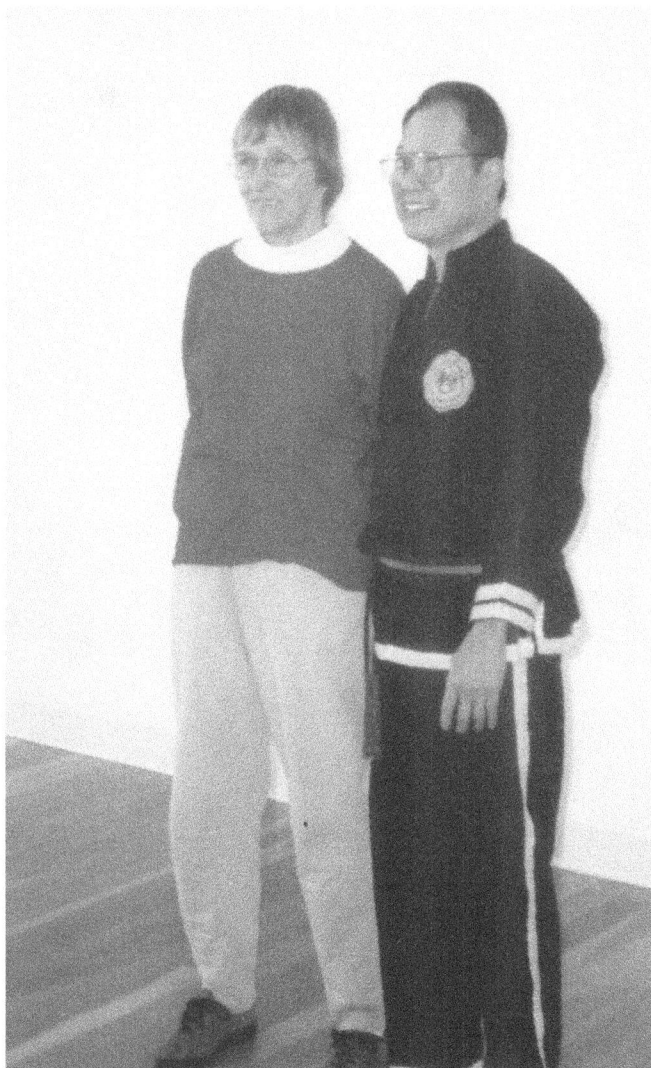

Joanne Von Blon and Grandmaster Wai-lun Choi at Twin Cities T'ai Chi Ch'uan Studio in 1998.

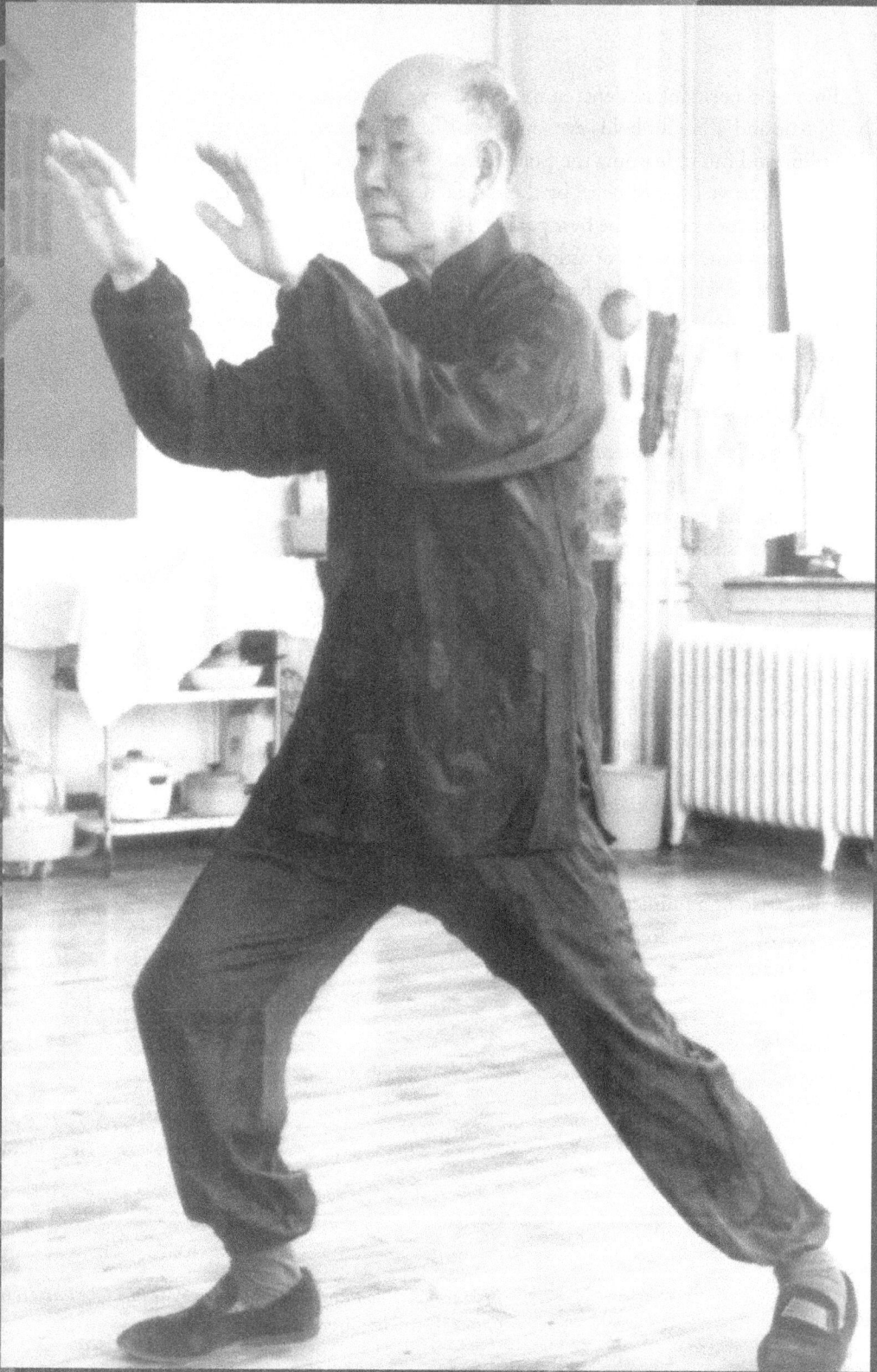

PAST

曙 ☯ 光

The year 2002 brought with it the death
of Master T.T. Liang at the age of 102.

This section contains essays written by Master Liang that will
continue to guide his students and his students' students far into
the future. It also contains several students' reminiscences of him.

Along with Ray and Paul's memories of their
teacher Master Liang is included a reminiscence by
their contemporary and classmate Paul Gallagher.

Opposite page: Master T.T. Liang demonstrates Push in his Boston, MA studio in the 1970s.

Why Should We Learn and Practice T'ai-Chi Ch'uan?

Master T. T. Liang

T'ai-Chi Ch'uan, commonly called T'ai-Chi, is an ancient form of Chinese classical dance created about seven hundred years ago by Chang San-Feng, a Taoist priest of the Sung Dynasty. The fundamental principles of this dance fall into four categories: health, self-defense, mental accomplishment, and the way of immortality.

T'ai-Chi for Health

In the Classics of T'ai-Chi it is said, "When the lowest vertebrae are plumb erect, the spirit of vitality reaches to the top of the head; when the top of the head feels as if it is suspended from above, the whole body will be light and nimble." This is the way to strengthen the spine, and by strengthening the spine one not only automatically strengthens the internal organs, but the brain itself.

The T'ai-Chi Classics also say, "The ch'i should be stimulated." The ch'i is an inherent oxygen in the body for stamina and vitality. The stimulation of the ch'i can be compared to the action of the wind on the smooth surface of a lake. As the wind moves across the water it creates waves, blowing them upward and downward in a systematic order of troughs and crests. The ch'i, latent in the body, is not sufficiently forceful of itself to increase the flow of blood, but if the ch'i is persistently stimulated, it produces heat and becomes powerfully effective in activating the circulation of the blood evenly throughout the whole body. The same principle is illustrated by the conversion of water into steam: the invisible power latent in water is made active and effective enough to drive the piston of a powerful engine.

If you want to practice T'ai-Chi, it is best to rise early in the morning and practice outdoors. If you want to rise early in the morning, you must keep far away from the alcoholics, the drug addicts, the gamblers, and get rid of all bad habits. Assimilate the new and excrete the old. Introduce rhythm so that the postures can be practiced to music slowly, effortlessly, and evenly, to create the coordination of body and mind. Early to bed, early to rise, a round of T'ai-Chi morning and evening, makes a man or woman healthy, wealthy and wise.

T'ai-Chi for Self-Defense

When you have attained perfect health, then we can talk about the second fundamental principle: self-defense, practical use. The application or functioning of T'ai-Chi hinges entirely upon the player's consciousness. It is said in the T'ai-Chi Classics, "Take advantage of your opponent's weak points and your own superior position." "Deflect the momentum of a thousand pounds with a trigger force of four ounces." "From the most pliable and yielding you will arrive at the most powerful and unyielding." These are sayings which emphasize mental activity rather than external muscular force.

As a result of practicing the 150 postures of T'ai-Chi, you will develop equilibrium (a firm rooting of the feet). From practicing Pushing-Hands you will come to know how to neutralize and yield; to lose, not to gain; small loss brings small gain; big loss – big gain. You should know all the techniques in the "Song of Pushing Hands" as described in the T'ai-Chi Classics.

"In Ward-Off, Roll-Back, Press, and Push one must know the correct techniques. The lower and upper parts of the body must act in unison so that an opponent would find it difficult to advance and attack. Even though he should come to attack with greater force, use a push and pull of four ounces to deflect a momentum of one thousand pounds. Entice him to advance; when his energy is emptied, adhere to him and issue energy. Adhere, join, stick to, and follow, with no letting go and with no resistance."

From practicing the Two-Person Dance (178 postures) you will develop an intrinsic energy in the sinews and tendons. This intrinsic energy is issued

Master T.T. Liang, age 84, demonstrates an application for Fair Lady Weaving at Shuttles on his disciple Paul Abdella for Inside Kung Fu *magazine in 1984.*

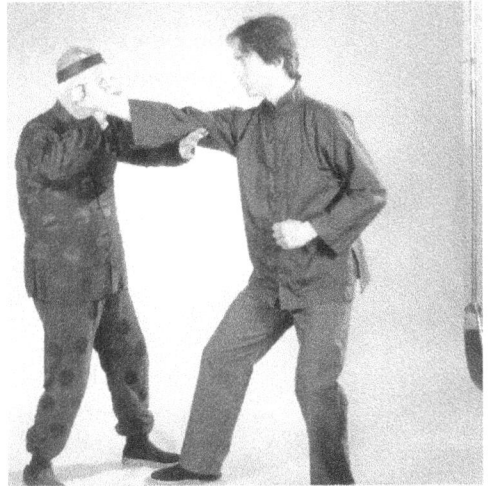

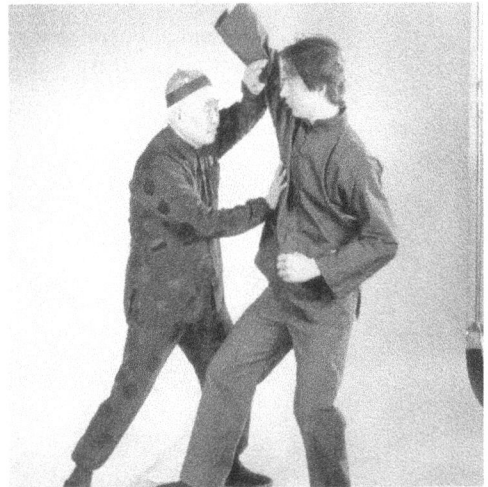

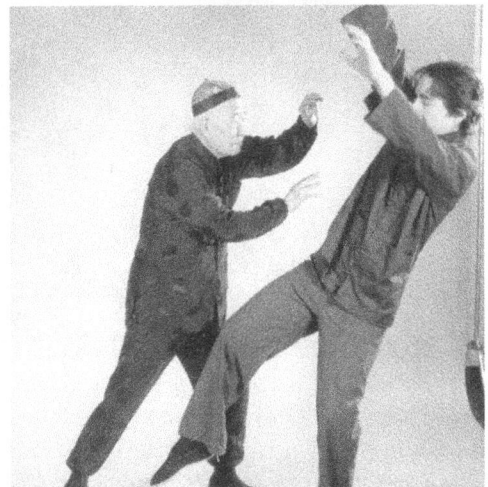

from the spine, the energy in the whole body acting as one unit. If you strike only with the hands, the energy will come from the bones and the whole body will be tense. This is not only ineffective for functional use, but also harmful to one's health. So the T'ai-Chi Classics say, "You have hands everywhere on your body, but it has nothing to do with hands." This is also the way to interpret energy. The T'ai-Chi Classics again say, "After you have learned how to interpret energy, the more you practice the better your skill will be, and by examining thoroughly and remembering silently you will gradually reach a stage of total reliance on the mind."

Eventually the "Sticking Energy" of T'ai-Chi will be developed. The "Sticking Energy" is divided into three levels — lowest, middle, and highest. The lowest level requires that one touch the opponent's body with the hand in order to make him fall — that is, one grasps the opponent's body or hands. There are two methods: one is borrowing his energy to issue your own energy (Receive-Attack technique); the other is to entice the opponent

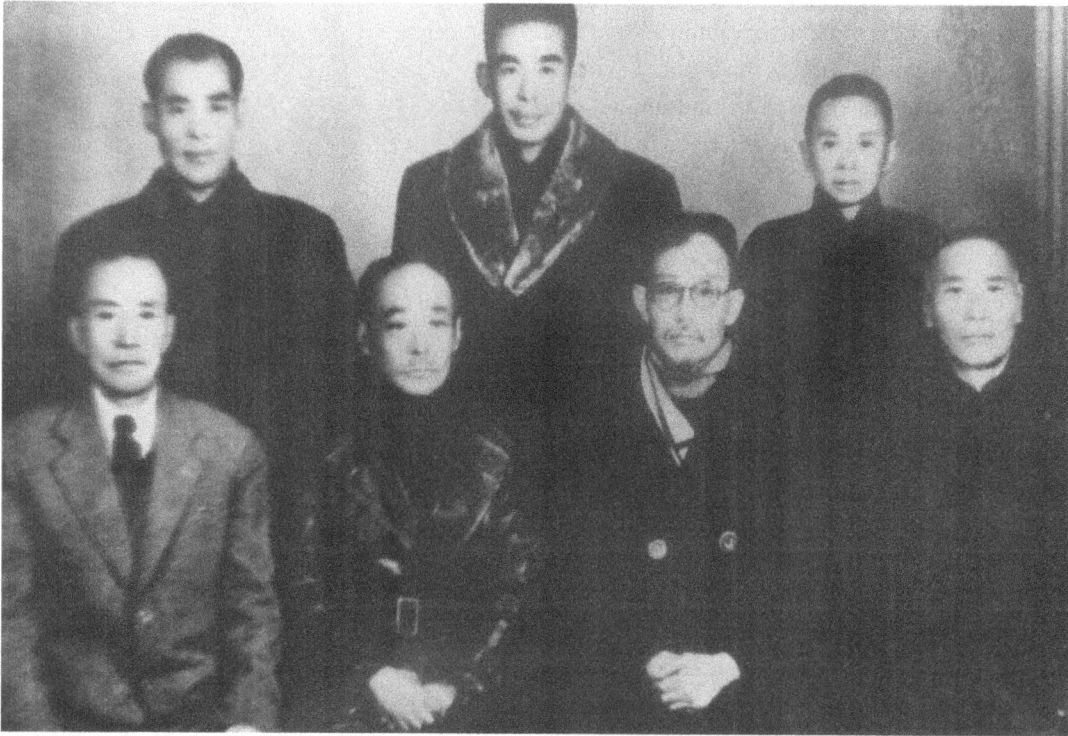

Grandmaster Chan Yik-yan (back row, far left) with his teachers; Grandmaster Wu Yik-fai (front row, second from left), Liu Ho Pa Fa; Chiang Jung-ch'iao (front row, far left), T'ai-Chi, Hsing Yi and Pa Kua; Chu Kuei-ting (front row, far right), Hsing Yi; Han Hsing-ch'iao (back row, center), I-Ch'uan. Two others pictured were not Grandmaster Chan's teachers.

to issue energy, then, after neutralizing all his energy to the side, to knock him over (Rollback technique from Pushing-Hands practice). These types of energy are the most elemental techniques in T'ai-Chi.

The middle level of "Sticking Energy" is described by the saying, "As soon as one touches his clothing, the opponent is immediately thrown over." That is to say, as soon as your palm touches his clothing then he is uprooted. "By touching the opponent's cloth, he can be overthrown in any of eighteen ways."

A person with the highest form of T'ai-Chi "Sticking Energy" can use his flat palm to lift anything, without exerting strength through the fingers. One of the T'ai-Chi disciples of Yang's family relied only on the sticking energy of one palm to raise an armchair weighing several tens of pounds from one place and set it down lightly in another. It is said in the T'ai-Chi Classics, "When the mind intends, the ch'i immediately follows." His palm was full of electromagnetism, like a lodestone, to which the armchair was irresistibly attracted.

My teacher, Professor Cheng Man-ching, said that he learned T'ai-Chi for more than seven years from Master Yang Cheng-Fu, the third generation of Yang's T'ai-Chi. Once his teacher told him: there are quite a few people in this world learning and practicing T'ai-Chi. They have to discriminate between the pure and the adulterated because like taking food, the flavor is entirely different.

The arms of a pure T'ai-Chi Master are like iron bars wrapped in cotton, externally flexible but internally strong and heavy. When grasping the opponent's hand as in the Pushing-Hands practice the T'ai-Chi Master's hands are very light but the opponent cannot get away from them. When he issues or releases his intrinsic energy from his spine it is like the bullet shooting out of the muzzle of a gun, swift as lightning, prompt and clear-cut like breaking a dry biscuit, without exerting the slightest muscular force. As soon as the opponent feels a slight stir of his body, he has already been pushed over more than ten feet with no feeling of any pain. When the T'ai-Chi Master only attaches his hands lightly to the opponent's hands without scratching or grasping then it is as firm as glue, impossible to remove and also causes an intolerable aching and numbness of his arms.

On the other hand, if I want to subdue and seize the T'ai-Chi expert, it is like trying to catch the wind and seize a shadow ending up with nothing at all, or like attempting to step on a gourd in the water, so slippery as to provide no firm hold or footing.

This is the meaning of real T'ai-Chi. My teacher Master Yang's words are so accurate and precise that I have tried them out oftentimes and they have proven absolutely true. I cannot but respect him from the beginning to end.

Mental Accomplishment

To accomplish T'ai-Chi physically and technically is relatively easy, but to accomplish it mentally is much more difficult. From my more than thirty years experience of learning and practicing T'ai-Chi, I have formulated ten theorems for my daily guiding principles to help me know how to deal with people and myself:

1. Nobody can be perfect. Take what is good and discard what is bad.

2. If I believe entirely in books, better not read books; if I rely entirely on teachers, better not have teachers.

3. To remove a mountain is easy, but to change a man's character is more difficult.

4. If there is anything wrong with me, I don't blame others, I only blame myself.

5. If I want to live longer, I must learn and practice T'ai-Chi and accomplish it both physically and mentally. To accomplish it mentally is much more difficult

6. I must learn how to yield, to be tactful, not to be aggressive; to lose (small loss, small gain; great loss, great gain), not to take advantage of others; to give (the more you give, the more you have).

7. Make one thousand friends, but don't make one enemy.

8. One must practice what he preaches. Otherwise it is empty talk or a bounced check.

9. To conceal the faults of others and praise their good points is the best policy.

10. Life begins at seventy. Everything is beautiful! Health is a matter of the utmost importance and all the rest is secondary. Now I must find out how to enjoy excellent health in my whole life and discover the way to immortality.

By learning and practicing T'ai-Chi and following the ten guiding principles for your daily activities, your hot temper will gradually become mild. Hatred, jealousy, anger, and all depraved thoughts will disappear and your evil temperament will be reformed, leaving evil to follow the good. Your mind will be upright and pure. When you arrive at the age of seventy you will enjoy a happy, peaceful, and quiet life. At that age you will realize that fame, wealth, authority, honor are all dust. You will then purify your mind and lessen desires so you can fully enjoy your life and appreciate Nature. That is why I say, "Life begins at seventy." You are wonderful. The world is beautiful!

THE WAY OF IMMORTALITY

The ultimate goal of learning and practicing T'ai-Chi is to become an immortal. Let me recount an old legend. When Chang San-Feng had sat in meditation on Wu Tang Mountain for many years, he still could not obtain his final goal: to become an Immortal. One day he got up and began practicing the T'ai-Chi posture, "Step Back to Chase the Monkey Away." After less then thirty minutes, he suddenly felt that all the joints in his body were widely open and his body and soul immediately took flight to another world (Paradise) and he became an Immortal.

Ordinarily the two bones of the buttocks are closed and the ch'i cannot sink downward. When Cheng San-Feng practiced this posture, he put one foot backward with both feet parallel and the toes of both feet pointing directly ahead with the distance between the legs equal to the shoulders, letting the ch'i sink downward to the legs and the bubbling-well points of the soles, thereby pushing the blood through the entire body freely and without hindrance. That is why he finally reached his goal and became an Immortal.

Chang Ch'ing-ling, 3rd-generation Yang Style Master. He was Cheng Man-ching's primary pushing-hands teacher.

The principles and theories of T'ai-Chi are so profound and abstruse and the applications so subtle and ingenious that you must find the absolutely accurate and correct way to learn and practice. If what you have

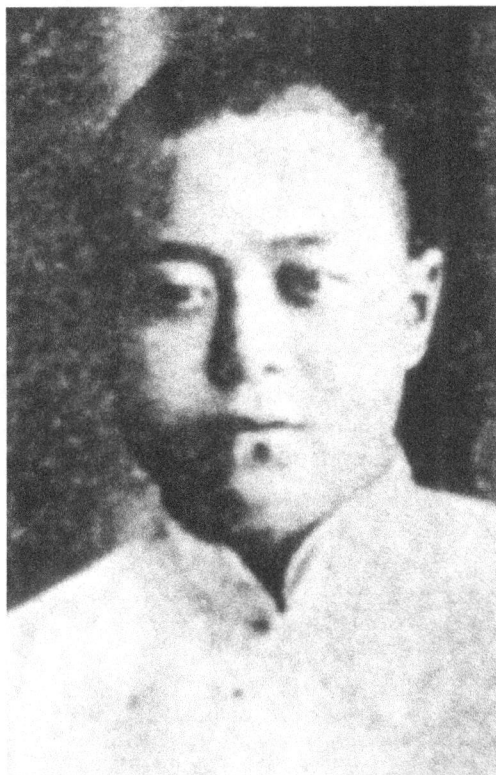

learned is not quite correct and accurate, the minimal error will keep you handicapped and you will fall behind by ten thousand miles. You will also lose the functional use of T'ai-Chi and it will be useless to talk about mental accomplishments and the way to immortality.

I have had more than ten T'ai-Chi teachers. From the point of view of his art, I must say that Professor Cheng Man-ching is the best. If you are one of his disciples and practice a formal ritual, you must closely follow his instruction when practicing the T'ai-Chi posture "Step Back to Chase the Monkey Away." This is the absolutely accurate and correct way. Whether we can become immortal or not by learning and practicing T'ai-Chi is not the main concern, but we have the greatest hope of reaching the age of one hundred years or more, the highest level of longevity. Nonetheless, a person's life and death are predetermined; riches and honors are in the hands of Heaven. I strongly believe in cause and effect. While we are living we must live virtuously, try our best to enjoy our life, appreciate nature, and finally wait for our allotment so that we have not spent the best of our days vainly.

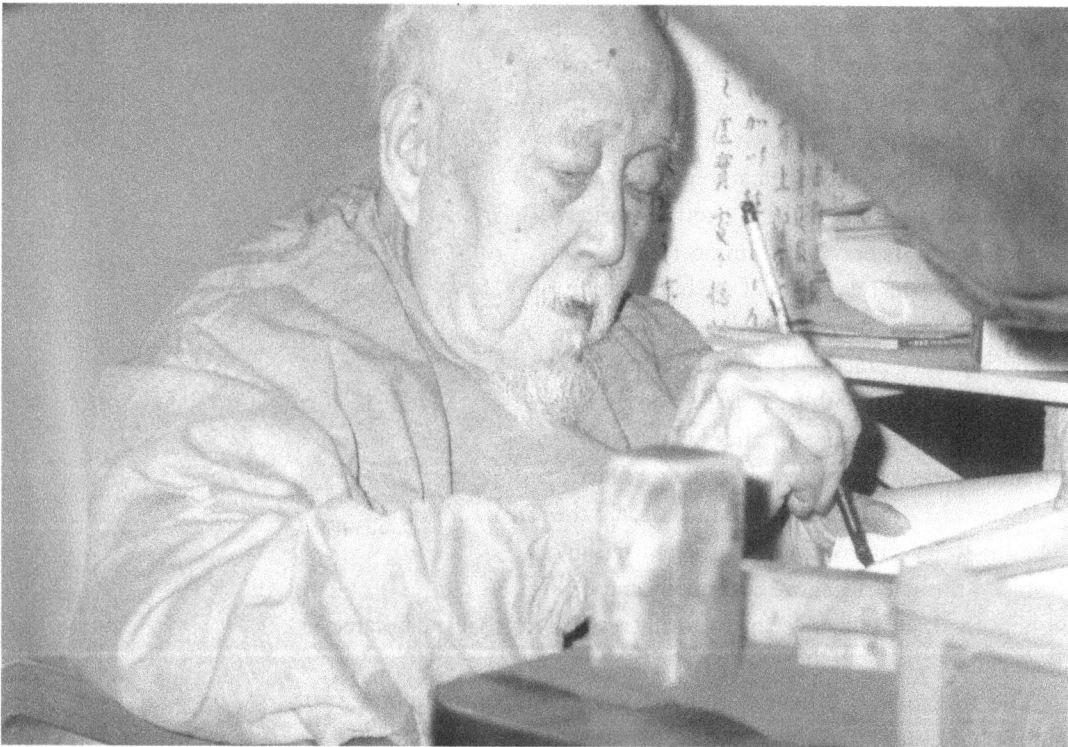

Master T.T. Liang practicing calligraphy in New Jersey in his late 90s.

THE COMPLETE SET
OF T'AI-CHI CH'UAN

MASTER T. T. LIANG

If you wish to study T'ai-Chi Ch'uan for health and also for self-defense, you must learn the complete set of T'ai-Chi Ch'uan. I shall explain the steps one by one.

1. T'AI-CHI FOR HEALTH

First you must master the 150 postures of T'ai-Chi. When practicing T'ai-Chi, you must follow the ten guiding points as mentioned in my book. To thoroughly understand the meanings of the ten guiding points is not an easy matter. You must learn from competent teachers, read really good T'ai-Chi books and comprehend word by word all the T'ai-Chi Classics which were handed down by the ancient masters who had already acquired this art. Only by following this method in practice day after day, year after year, for a long period of time can you finally enjoy perfect health and obtain a central equilibrium. This is the only correct and accurate way. So the T'ai-Chi Classics said, "The principles and theories of T'ai-Chi are so profound and abstruse and the applications are so subtle and ingenious that you must find out the absolutely accurate and correct way to learn and practice. If what you have learned is not quite correct and accurate, the minimal error will keep you handicapped and you will fall behind a thousand miles. You will also lose the functional use of T'ai-Chi. Students must heed this well."

When you have mastered all the 150 postures, you will enjoy a perfect health and obtain a central equilibrium and then you can talk about the second part of T'ai-Chi, which is for self-defense.

2. T'AI-CHI FOR SELF-DEFENSE

The aspect of self-defense is usually subdivided into three sections: pushing-hands and Ta-Lu, two-person dance, and weapons.

Pushing Hands and Ta-Lu

By learning pushing-hands and Ta-Lu, you will find out how to relax, yield and neutralize. The waist becomes like a willow tree, bending a hundred times in bonelessness. Learn how to lose, not to gain. Small loss, small gain; great loss, great gain. The most important posture in pushing-hands is Roll Back. When withdrawing your body backward at the last moment, you must turn your left hand palm upward. When you have mastered how to yield and neutralize, then you will learn how to counterattack. When practicing pushing-hands, my teacher, Professor Cheng Man-ching, often told his students, "When applying Roll Back techniques, don't let your opponent's energy come to your body, and when applying Ward Off and Push techniques, don't let your energy go to your opponent's body. You have to find the insubstantial and substantial, the center gravity, and the lines from your opponent's body (there are a total of 25 lines). Before attacking you must gain a superior position in your opponent. When attacking, the energy is issued from the spine, and the whole body should act as one unit. You have hands everywhere on your body but it has nothing to do with hands. All the abovementioned secret techniques were handed down to me by my teacher, Yang Cheng-fu." "If I do not tell you, you can never acquire this art in your whole life." I have tried and tried, and found that what my teacher said is absolutely true. After you have mastered the pushing-hands techniques, your intrinsic energy will be developed. Then you must learn the two-person form.

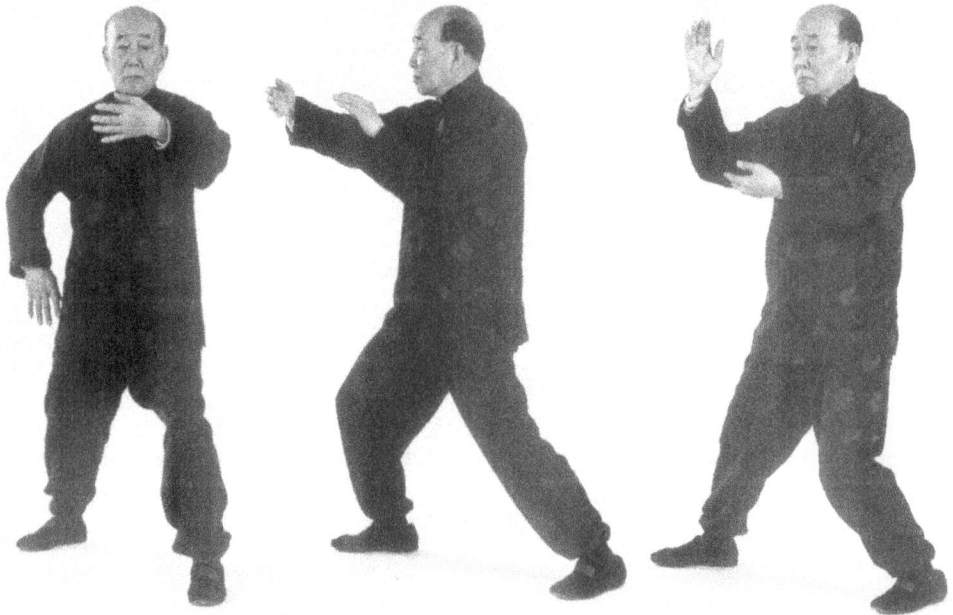

Master T.T. Liang demonstrates Ward Off Left, Ward Off Right, Roll Back, Press, Push and Single Whip.

String of Pearls

Two-Person Dance

The two-person dance (also called miscellaneous combat) consists of 178 postures, and each posture usually consists of three movements (neutralize, hold, strike). Let me give an example.

First Movement: When the opponent strikes with their hand, you must know the correct way to neutralize your body to avoid their strike.

Second Movement: You have to put your body into a superior position by adjusting your legs and waist and immediately hold their hand or arm, or lightly touch their body, in order to understand their balance of substantial and insubstantial.

Third Movement: You have to discover your opponent's defect, put him or her into a defective position, or find out their dead joints—then immediately strike. When striking, the whole body should be relaxed and act as one unit. So the T'ai-Chi Classics said, "The hands, feet, legs and waist must act as one so that when advancing and retreating you will obtain a good opportunity (from the opponent's body) and a superior position (from your own body). If you fail to gain these advantages your body will be in a state of disorder and confusion. The only way to correct this fault is

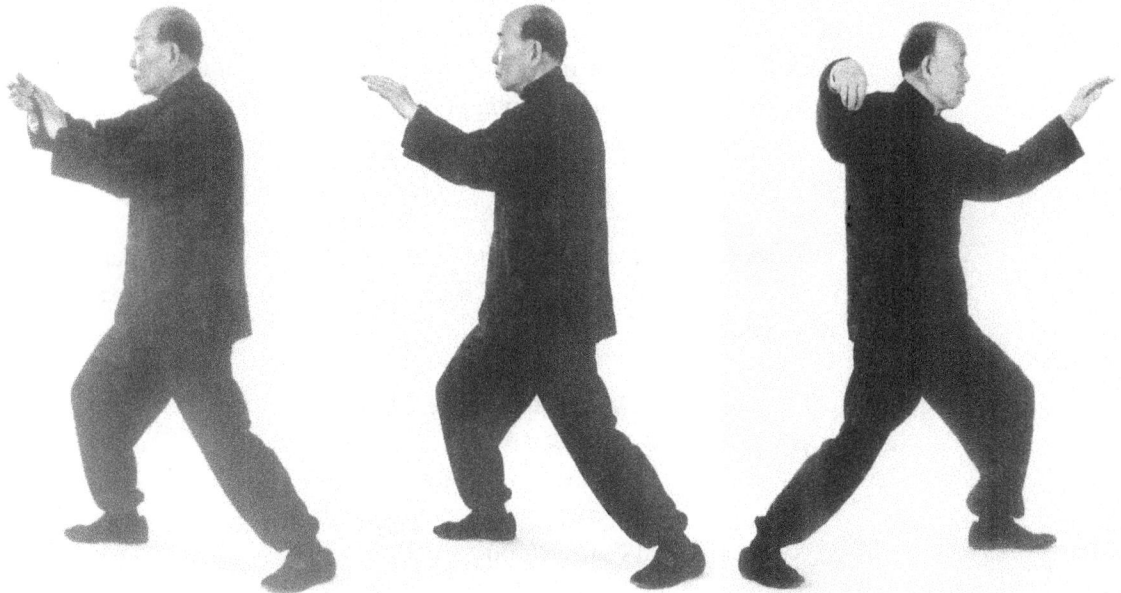

by adjusting your legs and waist." It is a dance when one posture is divided into three movements and it is a knockout when the three movements are combined into one.

When you have mastered the techniques of the two-person dance, you will know all the functional uses of the 150 postures of T'ai-Chi Ch'uan, so when you practice T'ai-Chi alone, you will have something to base it on in your mind. For example: When practicing the posture Deflect, Intercept and Punch, followed by the posture Withdraw and Push, you presume that when your opponent strikes your chest with their right fist, 1) you will neutralize and put your right fist on their right wrist with palm upward and your left hand palm downward on their right forearm and press down (Deflect), 2) step forward with your left leg and at the same time move your left palm to the forward left (Intercept), 3) strike the opponent's chest with your right fist with tigermouth upward (Punch).

In the second posture, where your opponent pushes your right wrist to the left with their left hand, 1) you will withdraw your body together with your two hands with palms facing you to form a cross (Withdraw), 2) separate your palms and turn them outward and then with your right palm lightly touching their right elbow and your left hand touching their right wrist, push forward with hands and whole body as one unit. (Push).

This is the only correct way to practice T'ai-Chi. If you have nothing in your mind on which to base your practice, your forms will gradually and unconsciously be changed to something different and the functional uses of T'ai-Chi will be totally lost. So when Professor Cheng Man-ching was teaching us T'ai-Chi, he often said, "When practicing T'ai-Chi singly you must presume that you have an opponent in front of you. This is also one of the secret techniques I learned from Yang's family of T'ai-Chi."

Weapons

After you have mastered all the techniques of the two-person dance, you have to learn the use of the T'ai-Chi weapons. The T'ai-Chi weapons are as follows:

1. T'ai-Chi Sword Dance (60 postures)

2. T'ai-Chi Sword Fencing (60 postures)

3. Wu-Tang Sword Fencing (100 postures)

4. T'ai-Chi Knife Dance (80 postures)

5. T'ai-Chi Knife Fencing (14 postures)

6. T'ai-Chi Staff (11 postures)

To practice T'ai-Chi without weapons is to strengthen the muscles of the body, and to practice T'ai-Chi with weapons is to strengthen the sinews and bones. When practicing T'ai-Chi with weapons, the body, the hands and the weapon should act as one unit so that the intrinsic energy will reach to the tip of the weapon. By practicing T'ai-Chi without weapons, your intrinsic energy can reach to a certain extent, but by practicing T'ai-Chi with weapons, your intrinsic energy will reach to the fullest extent and to the highest level.

How can you enjoy a good health for your whole life and defend yourself in times of emergency? Come on now! Let us learn and practice the Complete Set of T'ai-Chi Ch'uan.

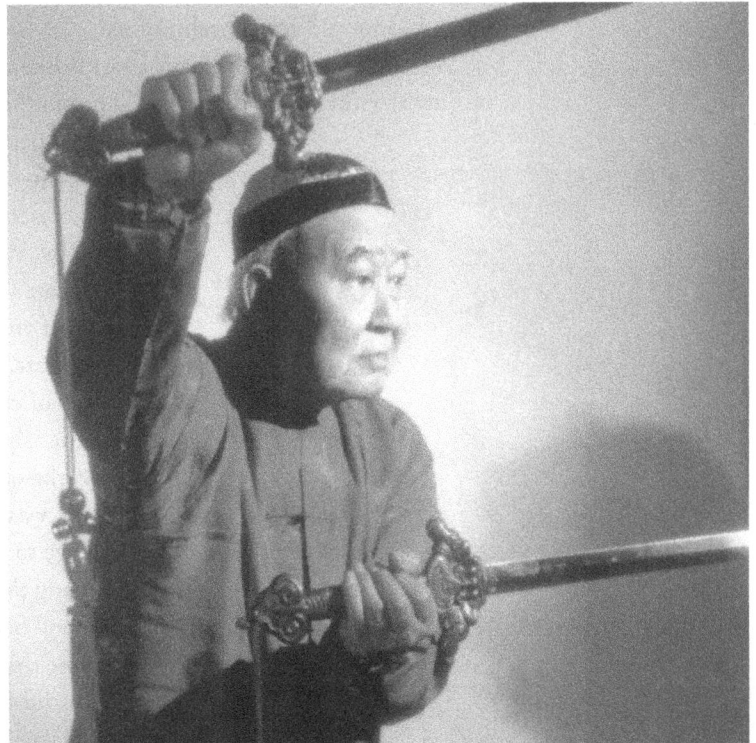

Master T.T. Liang with double swords for a 1984 Inside Kung Fu *magazine article.*

Why We Should Practice T'ai-Chi to Music

Master T. T. Liang

More than one thousand years ago a Chinese monk named Chan Chung developed a method of concentration during meditation. He told people to repeat silently "What did I look like before I was born?" … that is, "What did I look like when I was in my mother's womb?" Later this method was handed down to Japan as Zen Dao, using the question "What is Mu (nothing)?" for concentration.

We often say that a human's heart is like a monkey, jumping and turning around all the time, and their mind is like a horse galloping without pause. When one begins to practice meditation their heart and mind are fully occupied with short cut thoughts. When one thought is gone, it is immediately replaced by another, giving the heart and mind no chance to rest and concentrate. So monk Chan Chung used his way of concentration to cut out all the other short confused thoughts.

As the question, "What did I look like before I was born?" can never be solved, you have to repeat it over and over again for a long time. Gradually your heart and mind will become peaceful and quiet, and only one thing will be left to think of— "What did I look like before I was born?" Finally you forget even the words you are concentrating on, so your heart and mind will be all empty; your body will be completely relaxed; the ch'i will sink and abide in the tan-tien, and the blood will circulate through the whole body without hindrance. It is good for the health, and also the way to metamorphose into a Buddha.

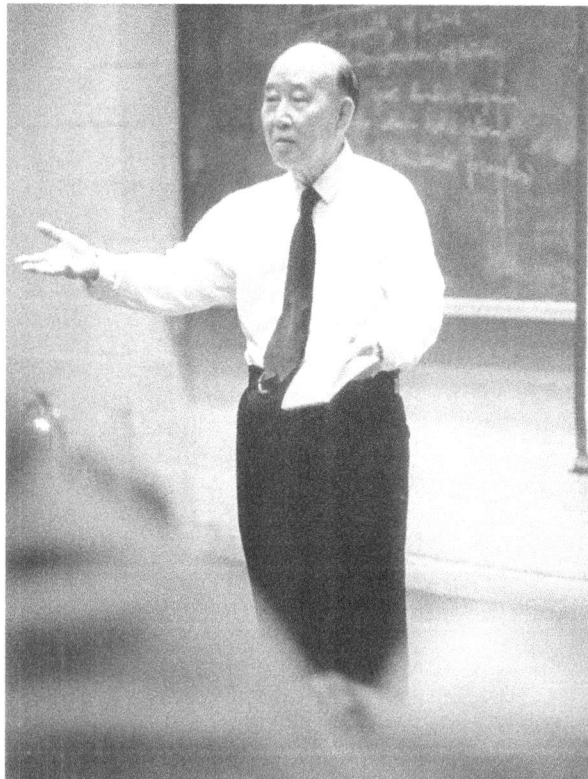

Master T.T. Liang teaching at a college in New Hampshire, possibly Cumbris College, in the early 1970s. He taught a one-year course there before moving to Boston, Massachusetts.

It is the same with practicing T'ai-Chi. In T'ai-Chi the ascent to the highest level is divided into four steps:

1. When beginning the practice of T'ai-Chi, you will have to memorize the number of beats, the directions, the practical uses of each posture and the ten guiding points as described in my book. You will breathe naturally, and will not use music.

2. After you have mastered all the points mentioned above, you will have to use beats, music and breathing (proper methods of inhaling and exhaling) for concentration, and get rid of all the rest.

3. At the next stage you will use only music for concentration and skip the others.

4. After practicing T'ai-Chi with music for a sufficient time you will forget the music, the movements, even yourself — although you are proceeding as usual. At this stage you are in a trance; your five attributes (form, perception, consciousness, action and knowledge) are all empty: this is meditation in action and action in meditation. When you finish and come to the end of the postures, suddenly you are back. Where have I been? What have I been doing? I don't know and I don't remember. This is complete relaxation of body and mind — truly good for your health, and also the way to immortality.

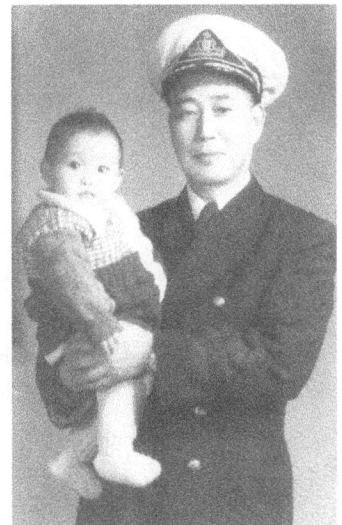

Of course if one can reach the highest level while practicing T'ai-Chi without music, so much the better. But I cannot do it because I am a human being, an ordinary ignorant person with a heart like a monkey and a mind like a horse. So I must use music as a means of concentration, as a stepping stone to the highest level of T'ai-Chi.

I have been learning and practicing T'ai-Chi with music for more than thirty-five years. After the first five years I thought I knew everything and started to criticize this man as no good, that man as no good, and to consider only myself as really good. After another ten years of learning and practicing I began to realize that I knew only a little. Instead of criticizing others I started to criticize only myself, because I was not qualified to criticize others

Master T.T. Liang in his Customs Service uniform with his daughter An-Le.

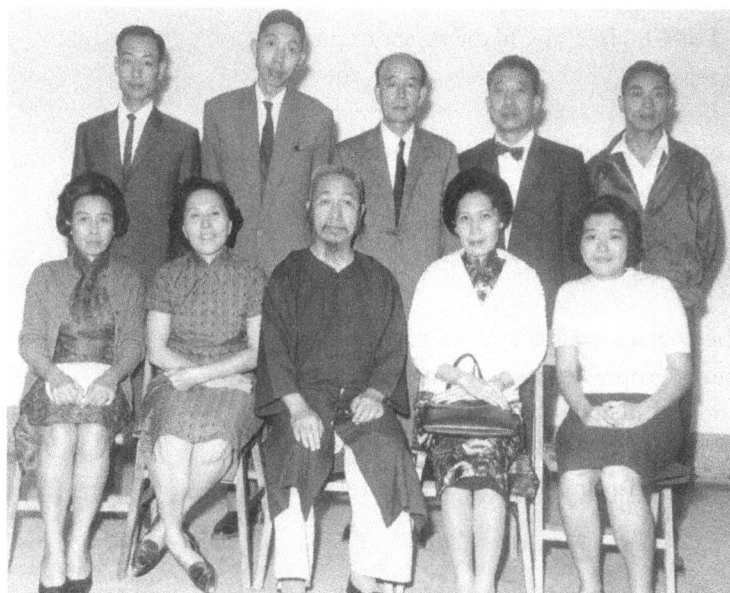

Master Cheng Man-ching (seated, center) posing with some of his disciples and their wives. Among them is Master T.T. Liang (standing, center), and Mrs. Liang Jou Shu-wen (seated, second from right).

with my superficial smattering of knowledge — and besides, I had no time for criticizing others.

After continuously practicing and painstakingly learning from teachers, books and Classics, and seriously criticizing myself for another twenty years, I understood that I was not qualified and dared not to criticize others because the more I practiced, the more I wanted to learn from teachers, books and Classics; and the more I learned, the less I felt I knew.

The theory and philosophy of T'ai-Chi are so profound and abstruse, and the functional use is so subtle and ingenious, that I must continue studying and practicing T'ai-Chi with music forever and ever. It is the only way to improve and better myself.

I like music, especially soft music, because it is in a human being's nature. It can relieve one's tension and anxiety, produce happiness and relaxation, improve harmony and coordination.

I have been teaching and practicing T'ai-Chi with music for thirty years. During these thirty years I have taught in many universities, colleges and high schools and have had thousands of students study with me. They all say that T'ai-Chi with music is good, and they have all benefited from it because they are human beings and to like music is in their nature. If T'ai-Chi with music were no good and were extraneous to the essence of T'ai-Chi I would have disappeared from this world thirty years ago. I am now eighty-one; I am still living and enjoying perfect health because as a human being I like music and have chosen to continue practicing T'ai-Chi with music to prolong my life.

A Questionnaire on the Occasion of Master Liang's 100th Birthday in the year 2000

What is your name?

Ray Hayward.

When and where did you study with Master Liang or one of his students?

1977 to the present at the following locations: Boston, St. Cloud, MN, Tampa, Los Angeles, St. Paul, Andover, NJ.

Describe his studio.

I studied in four different studios, so I will describe some common qualities. There were mattresses on the wall for Pushing-Hands practice, weapons and weapons racks, calligraphy on the walls, and the combined smell of incense, Tiger Balm and food. Except for his house, I was given keys by Master Liang to all of the studios and I felt they were sacred practice halls, imbued with the Master's energy, whether he was present or not.

Describe his teaching style.

Studying with Master Liang was an experience I have never been able to duplicate. Master Liang had so many teaching methods and techniques that it was like studying with Yoda, Lao-tse, Don Juan Matus, Bilbo Baggins, Bob Hope, Blind Master Po, Andrew Dice Clay, Yang Lu-chan, and the Buddha all wrapped up into one person.

No one, and I repeat, no one knew Professor Cheng Man-ching as well or as deeply as Master Liang. Professor Cheng was the consummate Confucian — very concerned with rank, status, hierarchy and lineage. Cheng bestowed upon Master Liang the rank of Da Hsih-Hsiung (Big Older Brother), which showed that

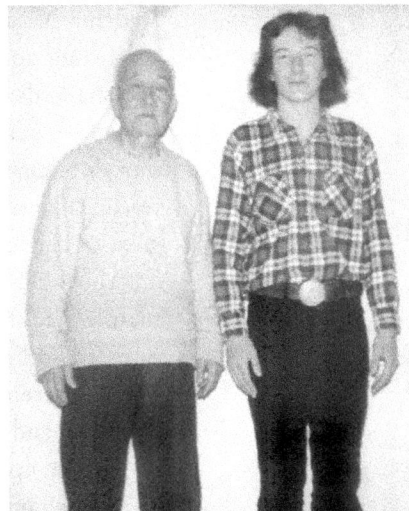

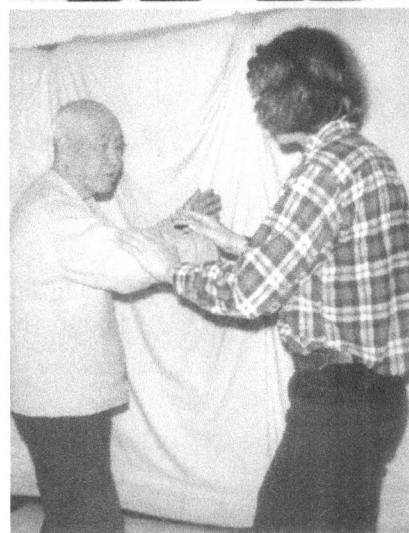

Master T.T. Liang and disciple Ray Hayward in November 1977, at the Boylston Street Studio in Boston.

Master Liang was Cheng's successor and had crossed a line of intimacy that no student before or after has ever achieved. Master Liang was Cheng's assistant, translator, co-author, and confidant. When Master Liang passed Cheng's teachings to us, it was as if the Professor was just in the other room.

Master Liang's knowledge of Chinese history, literature, and language, as well as British and American history, literature and language, gave many opportunities to draw parallels and make connections for his Western students. Master Liang used direct and indirect teaching methods, commands, intimidations, and used the "old-man" or "dear old grandfather" persona to the fullest advantage.

For me personally, I only wanted to study Martial Arts. Master Liang introduced me to more concepts, principles, and methods than any other teacher I have ever had. Only later in my studies did I find out what a great teacher of healing, meditation, philosophy, and life he could be.

Above all, time has shown that Master Liang's teachings are multileveled. Some of his lessons are like ripe fruit, ready to eat and be digested. Others are like a tree or plant that still needs time to bear fruit. And I'm recently discovering his lessons which were planted in my heart like seeds and are just starting to sprout.

To sum up: although Master Liang could and did use explanations, he also had an uncanny ability to teach through example, which reminds me of a quote from the Tao Te Ching which says, "Teaching without words is understood by the very few."

How many other students were in class?

Group classes were anywhere from 8 to 15. Private classes were usually just myself or 1 or 2 others.

How long did you study with Master Liang?

July 29, 1977, to the present. I always learn from him — every time I'm in his presence.

Describe a typical class.

Depending upon the subject, we would do 5 warm-ups, 2 ch'i-kungs and one round of the long form. Then Master Liang would get out his notes and materials and he would begin correcting, teaching and reviewing. In private classes he was my partner for all the 2-person training (a touch is worth a thousand words).

We always took a tea break in the middle, and here is where the old Master would talk, answer questions and tell stories and history that would hold us spellbound. Then he would look up at the clock and say, "Oh, I've taken so much of your class time talking about rubbish, so we will go over time."

Please recount a story that has lasting memory for you.

At one point, my relationship with Master Liang had gone from outsider to insider, from student to assistant, from superficial to intimate. One time, after I had made some mistakes, which I won't discuss here, Master Liang scolded me, saying, "You have disappointed me." I felt the very depth of shame at that moment. Then he said something that shocked me. He said, "But I know I've disappointed you too. What did you expect? Now we can go on." As I grow older this has been the definition of a functioning student-teacher relationship for me.

What is his distinctive contribution to T'ai-Chi?

Master Liang made the bridges between East and West, Chinese and English, old age and youth, sickness and health, mystery and attainment, and past, present and future.

What T'ai-Chi lesson has stuck with you?

Growing up in the Boston area, it seemed everyone had a scam or a con. When people would ask Master Liang for advice on a physical problem, a worry or concern, or some trouble in their personal life, Master Liang always told them, "Try to relax it." I used to think that was his scam answer to get people to stop bugging him, myself included. I realize now it wasn't a scam, it was simply that he had distilled the essences of T'ai-Chi, meditation, religion, philosophy, and healing into one short useful sentence.

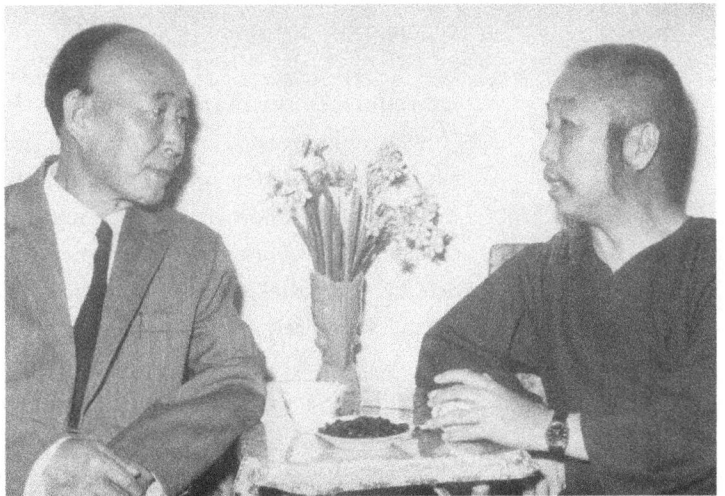

Master T.T. Liang visits with his teacher Master Cheng Man-ching in Taiwan in the 1950s.

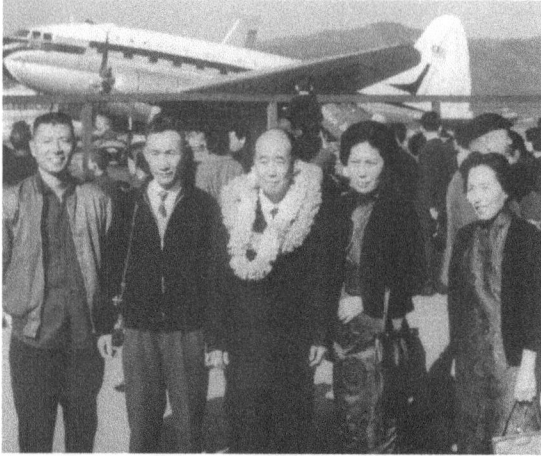

Master T.T. Liang at the airport with his wife, Mrs. Liang Jou Shu-wen (2nd from right), etc., before his departure for America in 1964.

How would you describe Master Liang?

I can only describe Master Liang from my personal view and understanding and experience. Master Liang is my teacher, my father, my hero, and my inspiration. He not only taught me T'ai-Chi, he taught me how to learn, how to teach, and how to live life. He introduced me to the friends I have to this day and the lessons I now give to others. He has truly touched every aspect of my life. In India there is a saying, "You can have many teachers in this life, but you can only have one master." I have had many teachers in Martial Arts, meditation, religion, and healing. Liang Tung-tsai is my Master.

What forms did you learn from Master Liang?

Besides the Complete Yang Style system of T'ai-Chi Ch'uan, I learned two forms and 25 knockdown techniques from 8-Step Praying Mantis. I also learned Shaolin Ch'in-na and various solo and 2-person weapon routines. Master Liang introduced me to other teachers to learn such styles as: Hsing-Yi, Pa-Kua, 7-Star Praying Mantis, Northern Shaolin, and Eagle Claw. When I met a teacher of Liu Ho Pa Fa and I-Ch'uan, Master Liang said these were excellent styles and encouraged me to pursue them.

Do you remember the use of music or chants in class?

Master Liang used exact counts for doing the postures and forms. He felt this kept everyone uniform for demonstrations. He also said, "When the form becomes consistent, the mind will relax." For the 2-person routines, the count let you know when was the attack and when was the defense. Only after mastering the counts did he encourage us to not use the music and rely on internal timing.

Describe the set of warm-up exercises and stretches you did with Master Liang.

Master Liang only taught 5 warm-ups and 2 ch'i-kung exercises. The 5 warm-ups are: 1. Forward arm swings, 2. Rub the kidneys 49 times, 3. Horizontal arm swings, 4. Waist rotation, 5. Toe raises and Push the Sky.

The ch'i-kungs are: 1. Walking Du-na, 2. "Cross Hands." Master Liang told us to stretch as much as possible, but he didn't show us any specific methods. He felt the form was stretching and more, so he used the form as part of the warm-ups for the advanced classes.

How did he influence your T'ai-Chi — specific examples?

Master Liang very rarely just told us what to do without any explanations. He would always give us theory, principles, and examples from the T'ai-Chi Classics.

One time I was given an old book on T'ai-Chi and I tried imitating the way the postures were done, which were an old style, quite different from the way Master Liang did the postures. Instead of telling me not to do them that way, he explained why he practiced the way he did and how the postures were modified and improved upon by the time he received them.

He usually presented his case with examples from the Classics, his many teachers and his own conclusions and then left us to choose for ourselves. From these kinds of experiences came a natural inquisitiveness and analysis that gave us personal freedom as students. Instead of becoming robots, we became researchers.

Many times Master Liang said, "Followers are dead. Only rebels can get something." This taught us to learn, study and research from teachers, but in the end make it our own way. Many times he pointed out that the different members of the Yang family each had their own way of practicing T'ai-Chi and that his teacher, Cheng Man-ching, differed from his own teacher, Yang Cheng-fu. Master Liang taught us that the Classics, theories and principles are constant and unchangeable, but what you did with them and how you executed them were personal.

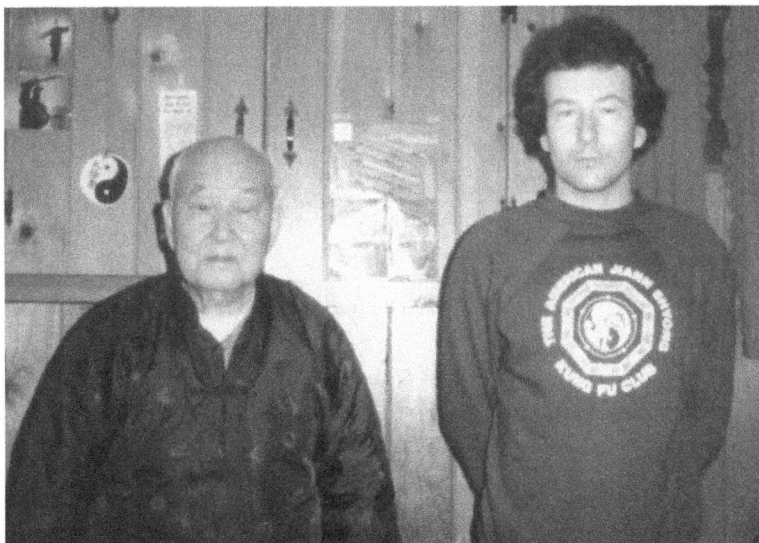

Master T.T. Liang and his disciple Ray Hayward at Master Liang's home in St. Cloud, Minnesota in January 1984.

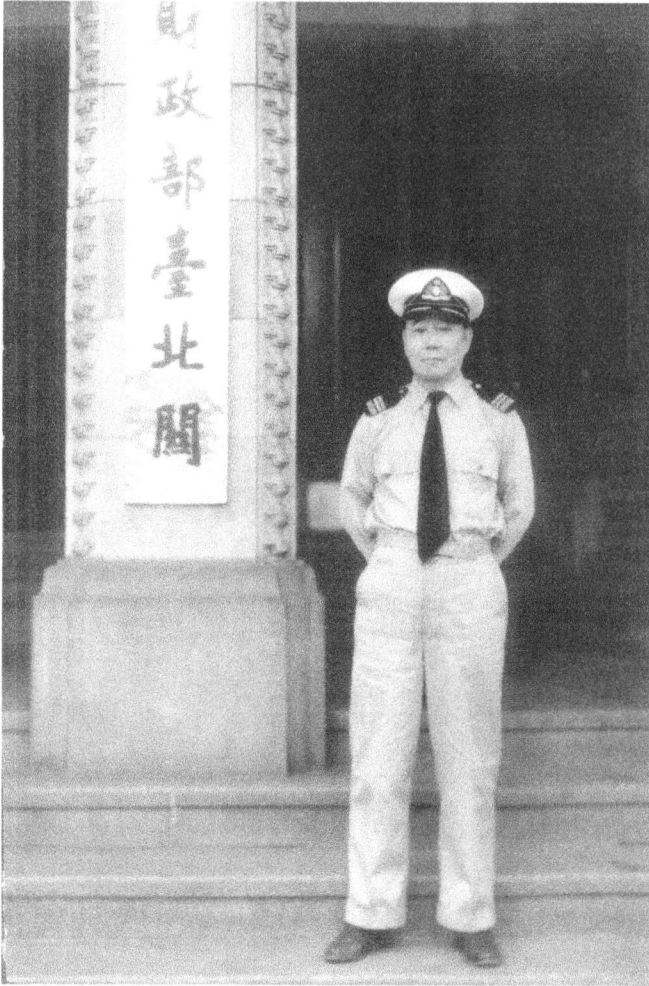

Master T.T. Liang on the day of his retirement from his position as head of the Taiwanese Customs Service.

What written sources do you know that feature or mention Master Liang?

T'ai-Chi Ch'uan for Health and Self Defense, by Master T.T. Liang

Drawing Silk: A Training Manual for T'ai-Chi, by Paul B. Gallagher

Imagination Becomes Reality, compiled by Stuart Olsen

The Wind Sweeps the Plum Blossoms, compiled by Stuart Olsen

T'ai-Chi, by Cheng Man-ch'ing and Robert W. Smith

T'ai-Chi Ch'uan: A Simplified Method of Calisthenics for Health and Self-Defense, by Cheng Man-ch'ing

Chinese Boxing: Masters and Methods, by Robert W. Smith

Martial Musings, by Robert W. Smith

Shao-lin Temple Boxing, by Robert W. Smith

T'ai-Chi Sword, Sabre and Staff, compiled by Stuart Olsen

Fundamentals of T'ai-Chi Ch'uan, by Wen-shan Huang

T'ai-Chi: The Supreme Ultimate, by Lawrence Galante

T'ai-Chi Ch'uan: Lessons with Master T.T. Liang, by Ray Hayward

Do you know of, or do you have, any unpublished photos or videos of Master Liang?

Yes.

Do you know of, or do you have, any audiotapes of Master Liang?

Yes.

What would you want to ask him?

At age 100, what is the happiest memory and why?

What is the one thing we should remember about Master Liang?

His 10 Daily Theorems, because they are the essence of the T'ai-Chi Master Liang Tung-tsai in his perfection (listed on p. 12 of his book, *T'ai-Chi Ch'uan for Health and Self Defense*).

Please add other stories here, while you have the chance.

Chapter 9 in my book, *T'ai-Chi Ch'uan: Lessons with Master T.T. Liang*. Also, there are three songs that whenever I hear them immediately remind me of Master Liang. They are: 1. *Old Man*, by Neil Young, 2. *To Sir with Love*, by LuLu, and 3. *Teacher*, by Jethro Tull. Anytime I hear these I am immediately transported back to my teens, soaking up the wisdom of the Master.

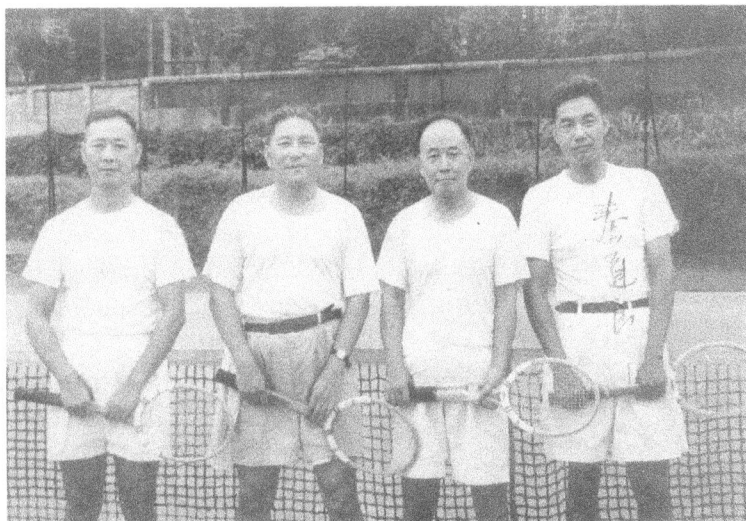

Master T.T. Liang (second from right), with three friends on a tennis court in Taiwan in 1956. Master Liang also loved to play soccer and basketball.

Master T.T. Liang—
A T'ai Chi Original

by Paul Abdella

I met Master Liang in 1982 when I was twenty-five years old. I had studied other styles of martial arts, but after seeing someone do T'ai-Chi for the first time just a few months before I met Liang, I knew I wanted to learn this strange and beautiful art. I asked around and a friend told me he had recently begun studying with a famous T'ai-Chi master named T.T. Liang who had just moved to Minnesota from Boston. My friend told me he would introduce me to Master Liang, and I could ask him if he would teach me. I eagerly agreed, and arranged to ride with him the following Saturday — the rest would be up to Master Liang.

After being introduced to Master Liang, he asked if I had studied any T'ai-Chi before. When I told him I hadn't studied before, he looked disappointed and said I probably couldn't catch up to the group that was already learning on Saturday mornings. I later found out that Master Liang had moved to Minnesota to semi-retire from teaching, and wasn't too interested in starting a group of beginners — most of the people he was currently teaching were already teachers of T'ai-Chi.

Still, I was devastated by his response. I told him I really wanted to learn and my friend would help me catch up to the group. Then I handed him the gift I had brought — a drawing I had done of a monk training in the Shao-lin temple. He studied the drawing, as I explained what it depicted, then he looked up with sparkling eyes and proclaimed, "Beautiful! O.K., try your best to follow the others." My heart jumped as I thanked him and I went downstairs to join the group. I didn't realize it at the time, but meeting Master Liang that day would change my life in ways I could never imagine.

Master Liang was a link to the past, and a bridge to the future. After his teacher Cheng Man-ching died, I feel he was the most knowledgeable practitioner of Yang style T'ai-Chi in North America. This was because he continually sought out the best teachers, and was taught by no less than seven direct disciples of second- and third-generation Yang family members. This allowed him to research and compare the techniques and training methods of the various generations, and create a distilled method that contained the breadth

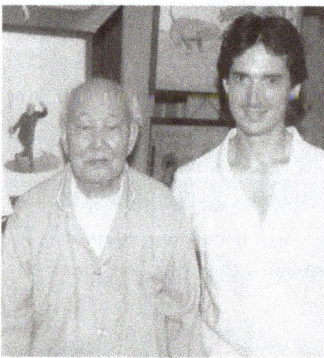

Master T.T. Liang and his disciple Paul Abdella in Master Liang's basement studio in St. Cloud, Minnesota, circa 1985.

and depth of several veins of the Yang's family T'ai-Chi. Master Liang was proud of the fact that he had had so many teachers, and had taken the best they had to offer to create his own art. "Take what is good, discard what is bad," he would say. "If I believe entirely in books, better not read books. If I rely entirely on teachers, better not have teachers. Become an incessant chiseler — never stop learning and trying to improve your art."

Master Liang did this continually, and his example became my inspiration. In order to master something, he made me realize one must do three things: imitate, assimilate, and then innovate. This process takes years of study and practice, but in the end it is the only path that allows one to develop an art that is both traditional and original.

Through Master Liang I have been given the gift of T'ai-Chi, which has brought me life-long friendships, abundant health, wisdom and peace of mind. More importantly, it has given me a means by which I can help others. I want Master Liang to know how deeply I appreciate the time and knowledge he shared with me and that I will be forever in his debt.

It is difficult to convey in words what it was like to study with Master Liang — any attempt inevitably comes up short. What follows is a brief description of my experience during a typical class in the years he was teaching in St. Cloud, Minnesota.

Journey to St. Cloud: A Class With Master T.T. Liang

Saturdays started early. On the road by 8:30, my classmate and I headed northwest about 75 miles outside the Twin Cities to St. Cloud, Minnesota. We drove through pine-dotted farmland, passing the exits to a half-dozen small towns along the way, including Monticello, where the nuclear power plant was. When we passed that exit we knew we were getting close.

Driving into St. Cloud, we passed the car dealers and chain stores that were crowding out the small shops that once gave the community a small-town feel. As we approached the one-story mustard-colored house where Master Liang lived, my thoughts always turned to the class that lay ahead. After we knocked firmly on the side door, Master Liang would appear and gesture us to come inside.

As we stepped into a small entryway that separated the kitchen straight ahead and a doorway to our left that led to the basement, the smell of cooked vegetables mixed with a hint of incense and liniment permeated the air.

Once inside, Master Liang would smile, greet us, and offer an observation. Typically this observation was limited to the obvious — "Oh, it is quite cold today," or "Oh, just you come today," if my classmate was absent. But it foreshadowed the keen eye that would scrutinize and monitor us in the class that followed. (For me, Master Liang's two defining characteristics were a disarming sense of humor and an ability to know people on a level that went well below the surface simply by observing them. All this while they were unaware they were being observed.) After our greetings, Master Liang would send us down the stairs that led to the basement while he returned to the kitchen to clean up after his breakfast.

This was the start of a weekly ritual, which for me began in April of 1982 and would continue through January of 1989.

As we headed down the stairs, we could see the rust-orange carpet that covered the basement floor. The walls were covered with pinewood paneling. The paneling also extended down two square-shaped floor-to-ceiling pillars. The pillars were spaced equally down the center of the room, creating three rectangular practice spaces. The first space you entered as you came down the stairs was the one Master Liang would sit and view the class from. The student in this space would get the most corrections since he was most visible to Liang. For this reason, my classmates and I would take turns each week in the front practice space.

The second space wasn't bad, really. It was about the same size as the first and only slightly obscured from Liang's view by the student in front. The third space we affectionately called the hole. Not because it was smaller and darker, and it most assuredly was that, but because the white cork-covered ceiling dropped down over a foot to accommodate some ductwork beneath the surface. This created a space that was not only cramped, but also occasionally dangerous. While doing a form that contained a jump, it was quite possible to hit your head on the ceiling, and weapons forms required humorous mutations on their intended choreography. Fortunately, Master Liang couldn't easily see those who were stuck in the hole, and in my nearly seven years of commuting to St. Cloud, only about three of those years required its use.

The two pillars, which divided the room, were branded with deep gashes from anyone trying to master a weapons form, and the cork ceiling held an array of puncture wounds that bled a fine white dust whenever you grazed it with your weapon. On such occasions the guilty party would stop and look apologetically at Liang, to which he would reply "Never mind!" as if to say "You aren't the first one and you won't be the last."

Along the far wall were two full-size mattresses stood up on end for use in push-hands practice. Next to them a long row of wooden swords, broadswords, canes and staffs leaned, one after the other, against the wall. Nearly every week someone would ritually replace a weapon after doing a form in a slightly askew position, causing it to fall over, taking the whole row down like long wooden dominoes. In the early days Master Liang would dryly reply to the sweeping crash with an, "O.K., pick up." Later on you were more likely to hear "banana head!" Then you knew he was starting to like you.

We usually had ten to fifteen minutes from the time we first entered the room to the time we heard Master Liang's slow steady descent down the basement stairs. This time would be used for some quick stretching and to review whatever form we happen to be working on.

Soon Master Liang would come down, settle into his chair and announce, "O.K., one round to the music!" We took our positions in our respective practice spaces; then the student in front would start the music.

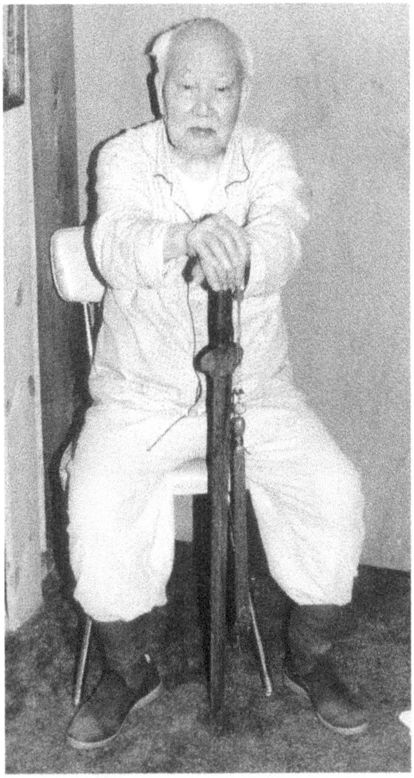

Master Liang sitting in his basement in St. Cloud, MN, circa 1986. He is wearing his pajama "uniform" that he often wore for classes at this time. The pants are tucked into his socks, which indicates that this photo was taken during class.

In the early days of St. Cloud, Master Liang would lead us in his five warm-up exercises before we did the form. These consisted of simple movements of the neck, arms and torso followed by two simple Qigong exercises. I was always struck by the short powerful waist turns that would propel his arms, free of all tension, into effortless, graceful patterns around his body. I would try and copy the look of his movements and would feel my arms begin to relax in the attempt.

Master Liang wasn't a tall man; he stood maybe 5'5" or 6". His rounded shoulders supported a round bald head with a wreath of fine white hair that wrapped behind and along the sides, framing a face that bore an uncanny resemblance to Yoda of Star Wars. When he smiled, which was often, you immediately noticed that all but two of his front teeth were missing. The two teeth on the bottom row were spaced apart, displaying an animated red tongue when he spoke or laughed. He had deep-set eyes with a spirited sparkle in them that seemed to look through you.

His torso was short and thick with a protruding belly he affectionately called his ocean of chi. At first this handle seemed an old man's idle joke until he allowed us to push and strike at his belly. When he used the technique of receiving energy, we were repelled backward with a jolt. This torso, however, made his legs and arms seem thin by comparison. He usually wore a sweatshirt of some kind and dark sweatpants with black canvas deck shoes. As the years went by, his attire became even more casual, consisting of flannel pajamas with the pant bottoms tucked into his socks, mimicking his elastic sweatpants.

As the music began to play, Master Liang would sit in his chair attentively watching our form movements. By the time we reached the first Repulse Monkey posture, his eyes would begin to lower and his head began to droop. By the time we reached Needle at Sea Bottom, he was usually asleep. At first we were surprised, then amused and finally relieved that our form wasn't under such close scrutiny. He would remain asleep for most of the rest of the form, occasionally stirring to bark out a count "3...4...da!" if our forms were out of sync with the music.

Master Liang knew every note of every measure in the music and where every count of a posture corresponded to it. If your form were off the beat he would wake and count aloud until you corrected it. How he managed to wake up just as you screwed up was almost as surprising as the corrections he made to the entire form after we finished — even the sections he seemed to be sleeping through. We never really agreed on how he did it, but the corrections were detailed and complete.

In general, form corrections from Master Liang were clear and direct. He would begin with a semi-encouraging statement such as, "pretty good, but not quite up to standard." The highest compliment you could receive was that something was up to standard. By this he meant it was performed according to the principles of the T'ai-Chi classics — the Bible for T'ai-Chi Ch'uan practice.

Next on his list of priorities was the music or the beat. "The beat is not quite correct. You must learn to do it to the music — to make it more aesthetic and more scientific!" Master Liang believed his unique contribution to the art of T'ai-Chi was the introduction

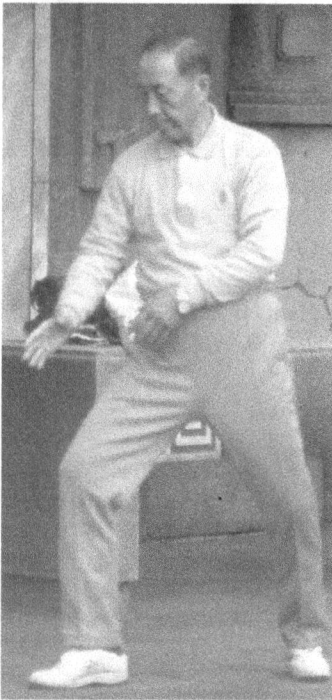

Master Wang Yen-nien (one of Master T.T. Liang's teachers) leading a class at Round Mountain in Taiwan in the 1970s.

of music in practice. He believed that in addition to its health, martial, and philosophical aspects, T'ai-Chi when practiced at its highest level was also moving meditation. In meditation, the integration of posture, breath, and a tranquil mind are essential.

To that end, the music — or more specifically the rhythm or beat of the music — was used as a tool to guide the body and hold the mind to a single focus, thus creating a meditative state. Nothing garnered him more criticism from his contemporaries and their students than the use of music. For the most part, they didn't understand his four-part method of using music to: 1. Learn the movements by counting, much like you would in learning a musical instrument. 2. Use the counts to follow the music and focus the mind. 3. Introduce breathing patterns or rhythms as a substitute for the music. 4. Discard all tools (music, breath patterns etc.) and just do the form as meditation. If they did understand this, they deemed it unnecessary.

Indeed, Master Liang himself has said in his article, "Why should we practice T'ai-Chi to music?" "Of course if one can reach the highest level while practicing T'ai-Chi without music, so much the better. But I cannot do it because I am a human being, an ordinary, ignorant person with a heart like a monkey and a mind like a horse. So I must use music as a means of concentration, as a stepping stone to the highest level of T'ai-Chi."

Often Master Liang would get up and demonstrate not only how to do a posture correctly, but how one of us was doing it incorrectly. This could be both humorous and painful. "Who is this?" he would say, making a face and sticking his rear end out in the posture Single Whip. "Is that me, sir?" I might volunteer. "Yes! You stick your bloody, silly ass out like Shao-lin. This is not T'ai-Chi's way!" He would then relentlessly mimic your posture week after week until you corrected the problem.

For some, this was not a constructive way to learn. For others, myself included, it forced you to surrender your sense of accomplishment. To realize that T'ai-Chi was a never ending work in progress, and that progress could always be made if you could set aside your ego and look honestly at yourself. This is not so easy to do. As Master Liang would often say, "It's hard to see the dirt on the back of your own neck."

曜 ☯ 尤

After the solo form and corrections Liang would announce, "O.K., what's next? Knife! Cane! Sword?!" And so it went, moving through the repertoire of forms that comprised T.T. Liang's T'ai-Chi art. In the end it was quite a repertoire indeed, with three solo sword forms, a double sword form, three

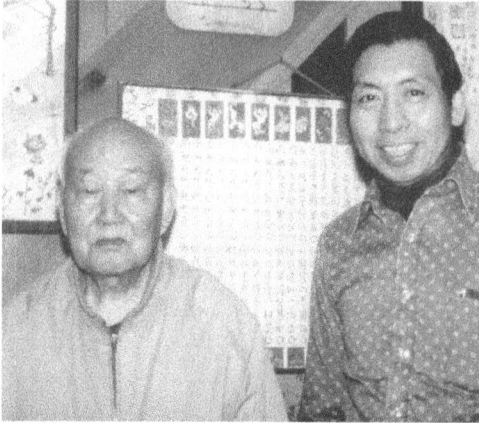

Master T.T. Liang and Master William C.C. Chen at Master Liang's home in St. Cloud, Minnesota, around 1985.

sword fencing forms, one solo broadsword form, a double broadsword form, one broadsword fencing form, a cane form, solo spear drills, two person spear sets, a two-person San-Shou form, push-hands and Ta Lu. All these practices in addition to the Yang style long form. It was a sink-or-swim teaching strategy that forced you to practice just to keep up.

When review and corrections were complete, we went to work on whatever new form or practice we were currently engaged in learning. Master Liang would correct what we had already learned then teach us something new. This part could be somewhat challenging, since Liang wasn't long on explanations. He would show us once and have us try, showing us again with some more instruction, then a third time before he returned to his chair and sat down. After practicing awhile, it was possible to coax another demonstration or two out of him, but not without complaint — "You bloody give me lot of trouble!" — as he got up from his chair.

Two-person forms allowed us to get hands-on with Master Liang and really get his feel — especially empty-hand forms.

After this instruction period, Liang would need to take a break. He would retire to a back room where a small altar held some fruit and flowers, two photographs of his parents, and a small bronze Buddha. He would light some incense, say some prayers, emerge from the room, and walk up the stairs to begin cooking his lunch. We practiced awhile to insure we'd remember the new material, then took a break ourselves.

Soon the scent of cooked vegetables began wafting downstairs. Boiled yams, carrots, lotus beans, brussel sprouts, and always cabbage — cooked in a watery oxtail broth to a consistency only a man with no teeth could appreciate. When the smell of lunch came downstairs, we knew Master Liang would soon follow to finish up our last half-hour of class.

Although many stories, jokes, principles and Classics had been strewn throughout the previous hour and a half, the final thirty minutes was where we would try and coax T'ai-Chi's "secrets" from the master. Of course Liang was never tricked by us into saying anything he hadn't intended to say, and often what he volunteered amounted to nothing more than idle chatter.

But those times when he sensed you had done the work, put in the time and were close to something, he would give you a gift that put your

T'ai-Chi in an entirely different place. Of course, he always let you know about it. "If I did not tell you this thing you would spend a whole lifetime and never get it." He was probably right.

Typically though, the time was spent somewhere between chatter and profundity with deeper discussions of the classics, and more stories. He told stories of the old masters, both his classmates and teachers, and those who came before them. Most interesting of all, perhaps, were stories from his life.

It was a life that began when the last emperor was still in power, and spanned into the age of computers and space travel. A life that succumbed to excess and illness, then health and prosperity. As a high-ranking customs official, Liang rubbed elbows with politicians, royalty, and criminals alike. He traveled the country, from the turbulent seaport of Shanghai to the frozen isolation of Outer Mongolia. He was imprisoned during the war and imprisoned by his vices, in time forgiving both his captors and himself.

Liang landed in Taipei, where he learned from the cream of Chinese martial artists in an era of great masters. Finally, at the advice of a fortuneteller, he ended up half a world away, teaching T'ai-Chi in America to a culture very different from his own.

I always valued my time with Master Liang, not because he was well known or he somehow fit the profile of an "old master," but because he presented himself as a fallible human being who shared the wisdom of his experience. It was the experience of a long and extraordinary life. Liang's art was subtle and internal even if, at times, he was not. This allowed it to get inside, to germinate and grow, not revealing a full blossom for years. But most of all, at least for me, his was a life that showed by example

Master T.T. Liang and an unknown man practicing San-Shou in Taiwan in the early 60s.

that what you accomplish in life isn't as important as what you overcome.

Master Liang went upstairs to eat his lunch. My classmate and I stayed behind to gather our things and write a few last notes. Once upstairs, Liang was already eating his vegetable stew, clearly more interested in his food than us; he barely looked up as we set a too-modest sum of money on the table for the day's class. We said our good-byes. "Thank you very much sir, take care, we'll see you next week." Liang, looking up again, sipped some tea and nodded. "O.K., bye, bye."

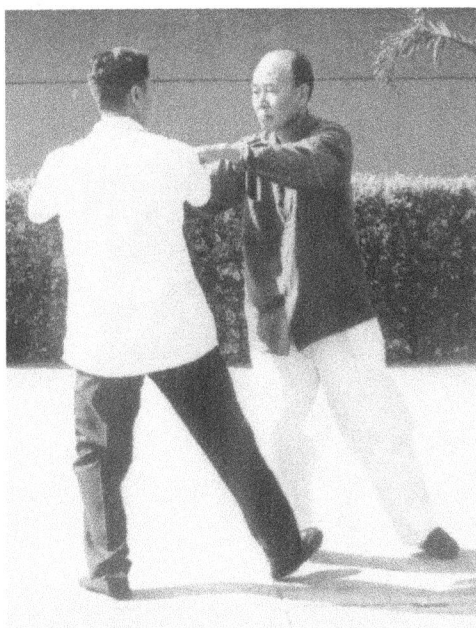

Good Health, Boom Da and My Students

DANIEL POLSFUSS

In the early 90s, Master Liang had already left Minnesota. Then one summer he returned to give a lecture. During this visit he stayed with me at my house for four or five days, and I was able to talk him into an interview. I remembered this interview while at his memorial here in Minnesota and was able to find the second of two tapes. Here is an excerpt from tape number two. As of this writing I continue to search for tape number one.

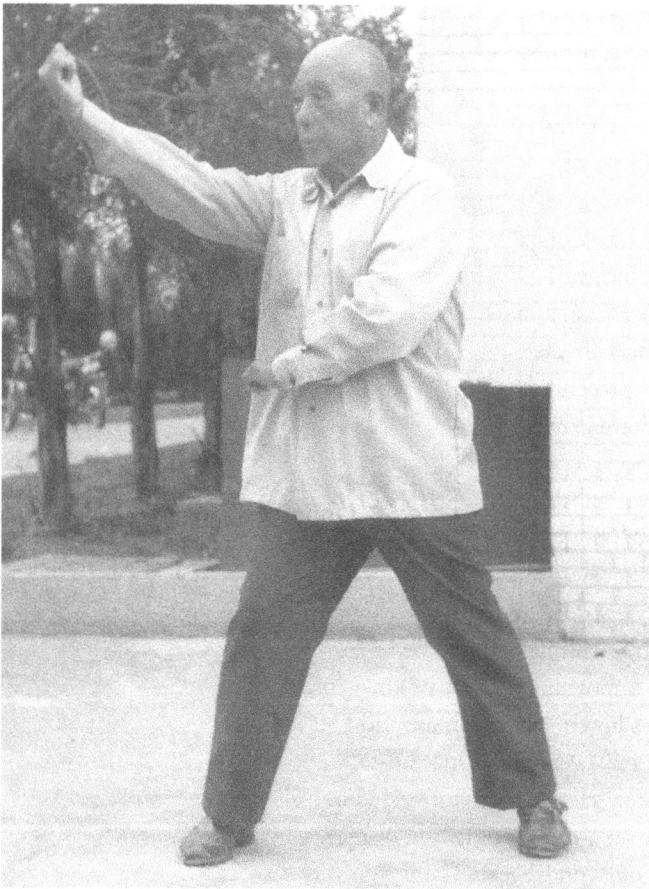

DP: Before T'ai-Chi, did you study other Kung Fu?
TT: Yes, Praying Mantis and Shaolin Style, many other teachers. After I learn from Cheng Man-Ching, I give up all these other styles...only practice T'ai-Chi style.

DP: Why did you give these other ones up?
TT: In my opinion the soft one not use too much energy...it is good for your health. To practice T'ai-Chi, you see, it's good for health. The others not too good for health. They use too much energy. (He punches out with a fist and makes a sour face.) For practical use it's all right, but not too good for health. So I want to live longer, so I want good health, instead of practical use. I give up all of the others, so that's why I'm still living.

Master T.T. Liang's 8-Step Praying Mantis teacher, Grandmaster Wei Shao-t'ang. This photo was taken in Taiwan in the mid-1970s.

DP: Please tell me some of the T'ai-Chi forms that you teach.

TT: I have this T'ai-Chi form, 150 postures, and this two-person dance ... with music, all with music. And T'ai-Chi Sword and Tamo Sword, all with music. T'ai-Chi Sword fencing, San Tsai Sword fencing. Knife, Double Knife, Double Sword, Staff, Stick. I learned all these things from different teachers. Making complete set of T'ai-Chi Ch'uan. I have had at least 10 teachers.

DP: Who taught you to do this to music?

TT: To music...I created this myself. With music it is very good for health, see. With music making you very happy. They like music you see. It is so beautiful, it is like birds singing. Make you so happy. You can practice, continue. I adapted all of these forms to follow by music.

DP: What about the beats?

TT: Yes, with beats.... Because when I was young, I learned dance. To dance you must follow music. Everybody do the same. No use to look at each other. You can do alone or with 10 persons and everybody does it the same.

DP: Don't you use the beats in a special way?

TT: Yes, use the beat like in the form you see. Slow motion, you use for T'ai-Chi forms. That way. Different speeds. Quick steps like the fox trot, you use for knife...then we have Man Jung Hung. So we have quick step and slow one.

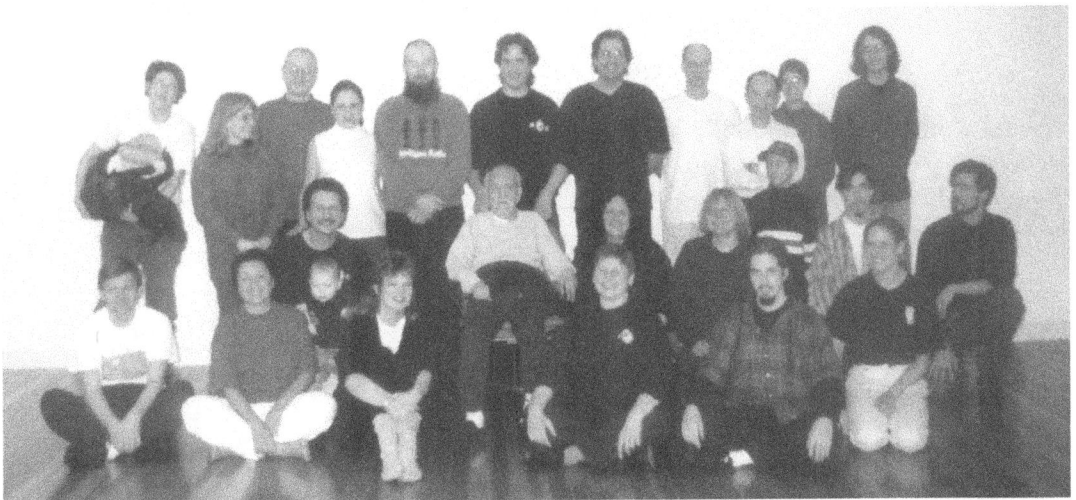

Master Liang's 94th birthday party at Twin Cities T'ai Chi Ch'uan in 1994.

DP: You taught me to use the beats as "Boom da, Boom da." Why do we do this?

TT: Yes, boom da, that means one beat. Boom da, boom da. (He motions a Press and Push as he makes these sounds.) Gradually you use boom da, but gradually you master it and you don't use it. You use inhaling, exhaling. (He motions through a Roll Back and Push, he exhales on the Push.) The four beats. In the beginning you use 1 da, 2 da, 3 da, 4 da. You must master this and then go to the breathing, inhaling, exhaling. First you must learn the beats.

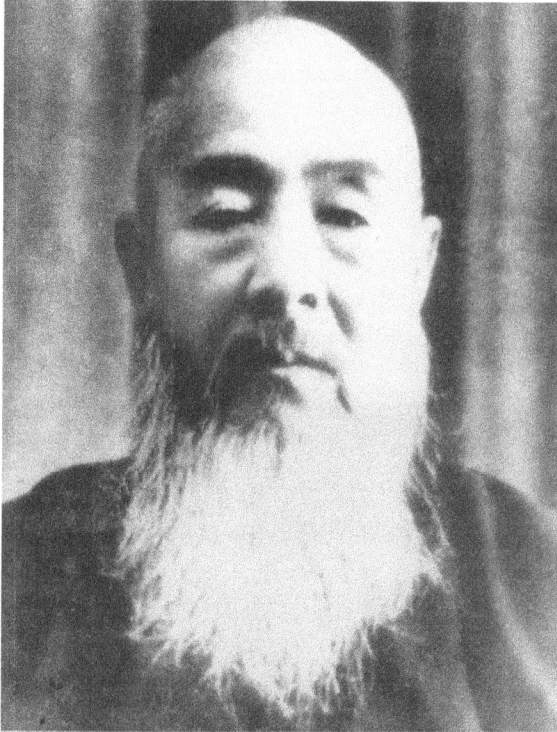

DP: Do the beats help you in martial arts...bring your chi to your fingertips?

TT: First with boom da, that means you withdraw, another boom DA knock down, that means you exhaling. Inhaling, exhaling.

DP: Is there one thing you want to say to all students, not just the good ones but also the beginners? Something that will help them to continue their study?

TT: All students I want to see that way. To continue study and gradually you will have good health. Thank you very much.

DP: Thank you, Master Liang.

Master Chang Chao-tung, 1859-1940. The Studio's Hsing-Yi and Pa Kua come from Master Chang through Grandmaster Wai-lun Choi.

Reminiscences of Master Liang

PAUL GALLAGHER, 2000

I met Master Liang for the first time in Boston, 1972. From the very outset, there was something about him that attracted me and that I later realized was a rarely encountered total authenticity — a kind of "root" into the center of his own being.

His teaching was always extraordinarily generous, in contrast to some other masters who would always hold their knowledge back. It seemed to me that he was utterly secure in his knowledge and therefore not the least bit reluctant to impart it freely — the only question was whether or not his students could "get it."

Aside from his very subtle mastery of the forms and applications, Master Liang taught — and continues teaching to this day — by the very example of who he is. And he is a master teacher. More often than not, his teaching comes in the ordinary moments of life, and frequently by his apparent teasing and bantering, which was his way of playing with a student's mental "root." He always seems to know exactly which buttons to push to demonstrate to the student whether he or she can truly "abide in the tan t'ian."

Master T.T. Liang demonstrates Brush Knee Left in this photo for his book, circa 1974. This was taken while he was living in Boston, MA.

Here are a few stories of meaningful experiences I had with Master Liang:

Shortly after I met him, I visited him and asked if he could guide me in studying the T'ai-Chi Ch'uan Classics. He seemed rather surprised by the request, but soon we were meeting several times a week and he was explaining the Classics to me. At that time, I was studying T'ai-Chi with another teacher, but had only the faintest idea of T'ai-Chi's application as martial art.

After a few weeks of meeting with him (and he refused any payment for instructing me in the Classics) I wanted to return his generosity and invited him to my apartment for dinner. Up to this time, whenever I saw him, he had dressed in a pair of sweat pants, T-shirt, and usually a blue wool cap. On this occasion, however, he looked truly dapper in a suit with

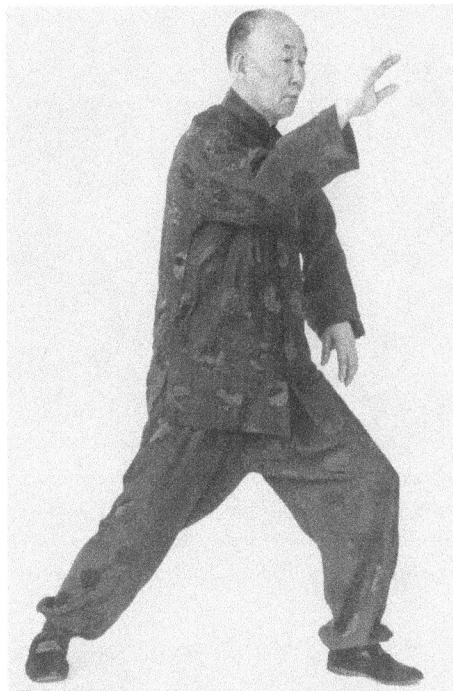

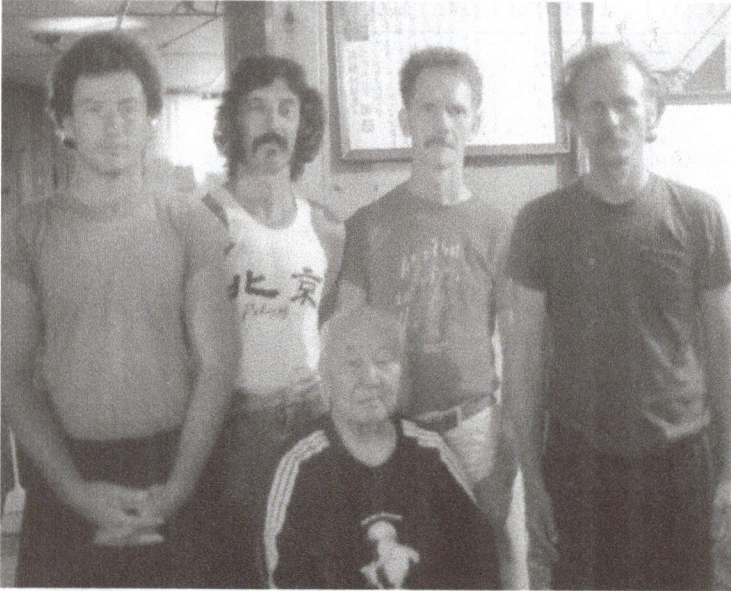

Master T.T. Liang (seated), Ray Hayward (standing, far left), Almonzo Lamaroieux (left), Paul Gallagher (right) and Twin Cities T'ai Chi Ch'uan's founding teacher, Jonah Friedman (far right), at Master Liang's basement studio in St. Cloud, Minnesota in the summer of 1985.

white shirt and tie.

As the meal was being prepared, he "casually" asked if I knew the application of Shoulder Stroke. (I'm sure he knew full well that I did not.) I mumbled that I had a general idea, but didn't understand it fully. He then asked me to demonstrate on him. "Come on," he said.

Well, I didn't know what to make of this, but decided to comply. Still, since I had been a weightlifter and Karateist, and felt that I was quite strong, I didn't want to hurt the old man. After all, he was 72 years old and I was about 28. So, as he planted himself in a bow stance, I hunkered down beside him and gave him a little nudge.

He looked at me. "Is this Shoulder Stroke?" he asked.

When I said yes, he seemed a bit annoyed and said, "Come on, do something." I wasn't quite sure what to do, but gave him a little stronger version of my Shoulder Stroke.

Of course, he hadn't budged an inch on either of my attempts. This time he looked quite annoyed and said, "This is not Shoulder Stroke, come on, young man, show me something." So I decided to really let him have it. I hunkered down again and thunked my shoulder into his side. He didn't move even a fraction of an inch, but looked amused this time.

"Very strong, young man, but still quite stiff," was his critique.

Well, it was time to turn the tables, so this time I asked him to demonstrate on me. He paused a moment, then agreed. I planted myself as firmly as I could, and the dapper little gentleman in the suit came alongside.

Before I knew what had happened, I felt myself propelled across the large living room by an unseen force. I felt like an old-fashioned cannonball that had just been fired. That was one of the few times in which I believe Master Liang really showed me his power.

I began formal study with him immediately.

On one occasion, after I had known Master Liang for several years, I went to his studio on Huntington Ave., Boston, to assist him with his book. When I was walking down the hall to his studio, I was surprised to see a well-known T'ai-Chi master from the Boston area leaving Master Liang's studio. I'll call him "C." Master C was a wonderful gentleman, about the same age and experience level as Master Liang, whom I had visited several times. He was well known for appearing frequently and demonstrating during Chinese festivals in Chinatown.

When I got into Master Liang's, I inquired about his visit with C. He told me that C had visited him a number of times in the past several weeks, apparently wanting to practice some Push Hands with him. This kind of situation would be somewhat rare among Chinese masters, so I expressed surprise. Then Master Liang said, "Yes, I can knock C down like a small baby." This surprised me even more. His comment seemed somewhat prideful, but then he went on to explain that C had practiced for some 40 years and still had no root.

As our conversation progressed, I was very touched because Master Liang, far from expressing pride, was expressing his sadness that someone could put in so much effort for so long and still have no root. He was genuinely regretful and compassionate for Master C.

Master Liang is an incredibly astute judge of character. One time someone came up the long flight of stairs leading to his studio. Upon seeing Master Liang, he said he wanted to study self-defense and weapons. (At the street-floor entrance to the studio, there was a large T'ai-Chi symbol with a photo of Master Liang and description of the classes he taught.)

Master Liang looked quizzically and asked the man, "You want to study self-defense?" The man said yes. Master Liang said, "You must ask the Big Boss. Big Boss is not here now …"

The man appeared quite confused. "You're the guy, aren't you? That's your picture downstairs."

"No," said Master Liang, "that picture is Big Boss. Big Boss is not here."

The man seemed bewildered, looked at me, looked at Master Liang, shrugged his shoulders and left. I was quite bewildered myself.

After the man's footsteps had receded down the long flight of stairs, a sly grin crept over Master Liang's face. "That man has a black heart. I can teach him nothing."

瞱 ☯ 光

Master Liang has always been a jokester, but it took me quite a while to realize the jokes have method in their madness. For a period of time in Boston, my former wife would drop me off at the downtown studio, go shopping, and pick me up after the class. When she showed up in the studio, there would usually be some bantering.

I often did not practice my form to music at home, even though I always attempted it in class. I knew quite well that Master Liang could see that much of the time, I wasn't quite on the beat when I did my form in front of him. So he called me "Big Rebel," and often asked why I didn't practice regularly to the music.

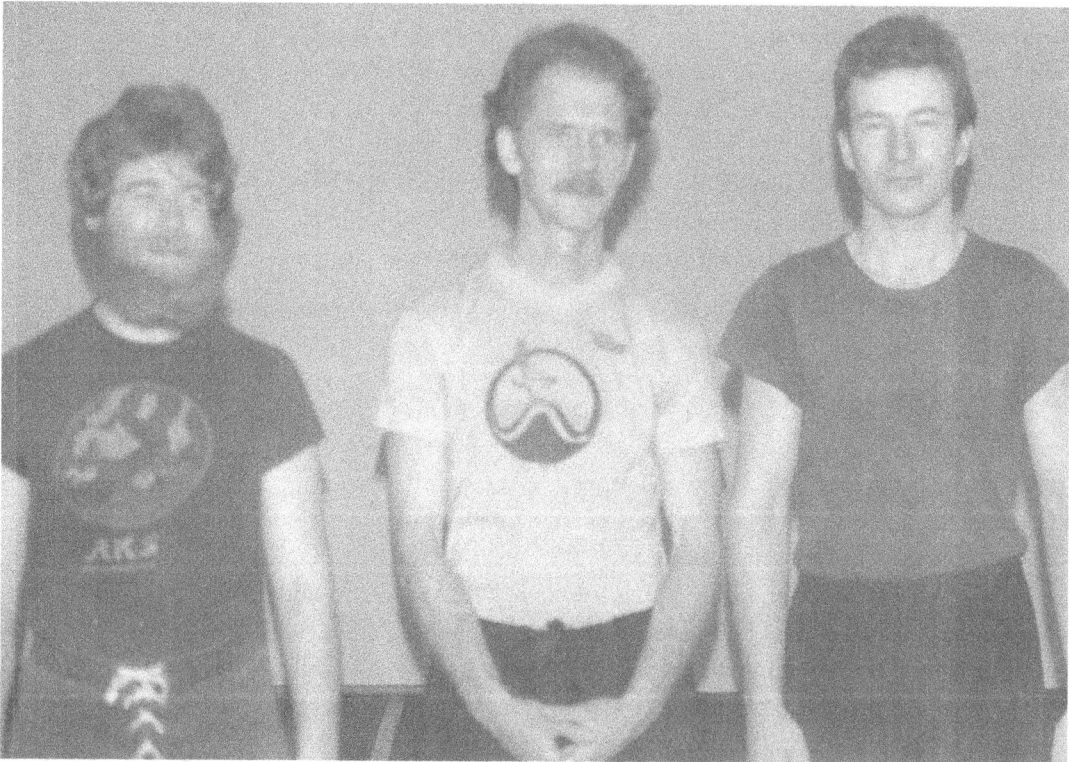

J. Richard Roy (left), Paul Gallagher (center) and Ray Hayward (right) at J.R. Roy's studio in Greenfield, Massachusetts in 1982.

On this occasion, when my wife came in, Master Liang asked her, "Why doesn't your husband practice T'ai-Chi to music?" She looked at him, smiled, and said, "Because he's stupid." Master Liang laughed uproariously, and I laughed myself. It was a joke and I certainly took it as such.

Years later, after she and I had long been divorced, Master Liang one day surprised me by asking if I remembered that little episode. When I said yes, he surprised me even more by saying, "I knew you and your wife would divorce; she did not respect you."

That really blew me away — I thought Master Liang had been checking me out when he asked her that question. In reality, he had been checking her out as well.

☯

Saturday mornings were the time when Master Liang's "old timers" would gather for Push Hands at the Boston studio. There would be old mattresses gathered from Salvation Army on the walls, so you could stay relaxed during Push Hands, not stiffening up in fear of getting blasted into a bare wall.

This Saturday Master Liang was impassively reading the newspaper while his advanced students were pushing hands. Some time went by and Master Liang continued reading the paper, even though this was supposed to be class time. After about half an hour, I went over to Master Liang and asked when he would begin teaching. He lowered his newspaper.

"All wild bulls, I can teach nothing …" and raised his paper again.

☯

I truly believe that Master Liang has changed many lives (perhaps hundreds, or even thousands) for the better. He is a rare and authentic teacher and his real teaching could reach the center of someone's being — going far far beyond mere forms and exercises. All of this was done in a kind of nonchalant way with the frequent joking, teasing, or seemingly irrelevant comments whose real meaning and profound application to one's life would only be discovered later.

If you take into account the "ripple effect" in which some of the essence of Master Liang's spirit and teaching influence his students, their students, and now a third generation of students, plus all of their families and the people they encounter in everyday life, Master Liang's influence is truly incalculable. He is truly a rare and special "T'ai-Chi Immortal" who continues each day to "win the last bout."

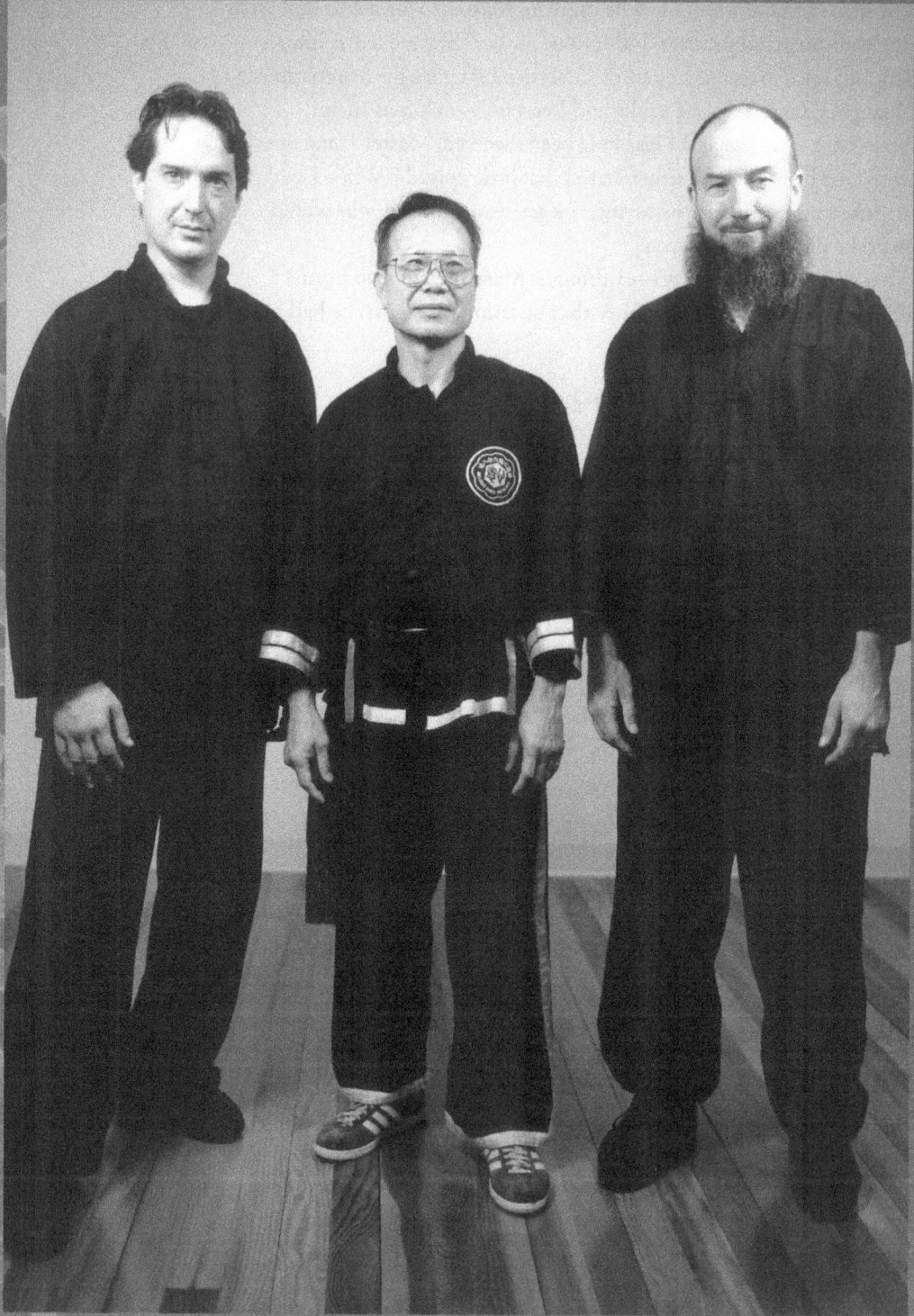

PRESENT

曙 ☯ 光

The present heads of Master T.T. Liang's T'ai-Chi lineage are Ray Hayward (Shu Kuang) and Paul Abdella (Huei Ming), the instructors at Twin Cities T'ai-Chi Ch'uan. Master Liang named them his disciples on November 11th, 1988, making them the sixth generation in the lineage.

Contained in this section are essays by Ray and Paul on T'ai-Chi and other aspects of martial arts, most of which have been previously published in the studio newsletter Wu Dang.

Also reprinted here with special permission is a treatise on Liu Ho Pa Fa by Grandmaster Wai-lun Choi, the designated grandmaster of the style. Ray and Paul continue to visit Master Choi's studio in Chicago to receive his teachings in Liu Ho Pa Fa and other styles.

Opposite page: Paul Abdella (left), Grandmaster Wai-lun Choi (center) and Ray Hayward (right) in 1996.

A Brief Introduction to the Evolution of the 150-Posture Solo Form

Ray Hayward

All styles of T'ai-Chi can ultimately trace their forms to the Chen Family style of martial arts. The historical founder of this style, Chen Wan-ting, was a general during the Ming dynasty. Through his involvement in the military, he was particularly interested in spear and empty-hand fighting techniques and training methods. When he retired, he spent his time practicing, researching, and teaching his three lifelong pursuits: the spear, empty-hand fighting, and Taoist meditation.

Chen is credited with creating seven empty-hand routines, which embraced characteristics of Taoism, and two styles of spear fencing. The first five routines of empty-hand were very short and were called simply routine number one, routine number two, and so on to routine number five. The last two routines were longer and were named P'ao-Chui (Cannon Hammer/Fist) and Chang Ch'uan (Long Fist). Chen used the theory of yin and yang to train the body for speed, power, offense, defense, and sensitivity. He added the ch'i circulation of Taoist meditation to calm the students' minds and refine their energy.

The first five routines were practiced with a ratio of 80% soft and slow movements and 20% hard and fast movements. This helped students learn defense (hua). The Cannon Fist routine, which has 72 postures, was practiced with a ratio of 80% hard and fast movements and 20% slow and soft movements. This helped the students learn attacking (da). The Long Fist routine, which has 108 postures, was evenly balanced with 50% hard and fast and 50% slow and soft. This helped the students learn seizing (na).

Gradually the successive Chen generations combined the five short routines into one long routine with anywhere from 88 to 108 to 150 postures called Lao-Chia, or Old Frame. This is one of the forms the founder of our style, Yang Lu-chan, learned and subsequently modified and improved to be known as the T'ai-Chi Ch'uan most people practice in the world today. When we look at the Lao-chia (we call it Solo Form) we can easily see the five ideas behind the original five routines.

Our teacher, Master T.T. Liang, told us that each of the original five routines began with Grasp Sparrow's Tail and Single Whip and ended with Cross Hands and Conclusion. Liang broke down our Solo Form into six sections, capsulizing the original five routines.

They are as follows:

+ First Section: postures 1-22

+ Repulse Monkey section: postures 23-54

+ Kick section: postures 55-73

+ Fair Lady section: postures 74-106

+ Repulse Monkey section (repeat): postures 107-132

+ Last Section: postures 133-150

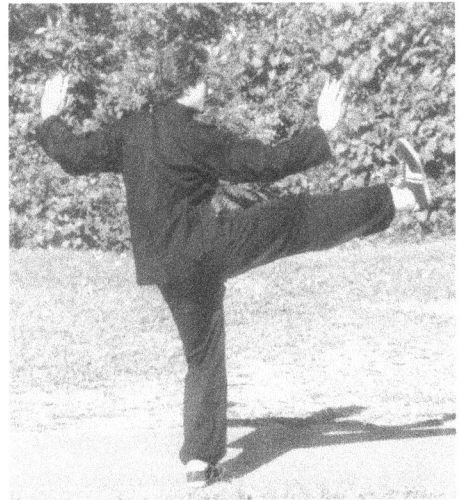

Ray Hayward demonstrates Turn and Kick with Sole on Labor Day, 1984 at River Flats Park in Minneapolis, Minnesota.

Each section/routine has its own unique flavor and emphasis, as well as its difficulties and lessons. The mastery in linking the sections together has held T'ai-Chi enthusiasts captive for years. Whether it was done intuitively or deliberately, the Solo Form sequence is a treasure of choreography that will bear fruit for generations to come. As this is only a brief introduction, I'll end here, but I'd like to share two quotes from my T'ai-Chi teachers.

Yang Chien-hou (2nd Generation) had his soft and hard in perfect coordination. So his Solo Form was yin and yang, soft outside, hard inside. Slow in practice, fast in use. Soft for defense, hard for offense. Because of him, we use only one form to practice all the variations of yin and yang.
~ *Master T.T. Liang*

Yang style T'ai-Chi is like a shark swimming through the water, slowly and smoothly hunting for food. When it sees a fish it moves quickly, powerfully, and attacks and eats it.
~ *Master Wai-lun Choi*

THE EVOLUTION OF PRACTICE

PAUL ABDELLA

The study and practice of T'ai-Chi Ch'uan from beginning to advanced levels evolves naturally in three distinct phases. The first is the stage of imitation, the second is the stage of assimilation, and third is the stage of innovation. To recognize each stage and allow it to develop and evolve naturally from one into the next is the way to cultivate depth and mastery in T'ai-Chi.

IMITATION: 1. TO SEEK TO FOLLOW THE EXAMPLE OF. 2. TO MIMIC. 3. TO REPRODUCE IN FORM AND CONTENT.

Imitation is the most primal form of learning we know. From the first utterances of speech to our first walking steps, humans have always learned by imitating the world around them. We awaken these innate human functions by imitating through sight, sound, touch and our other senses. Through imitation and the assistance of our caregivers, we acquire the ability to walk, talk, feed and dress ourselves and to perform other basic life skills.

As we mature, we cultivate interests and seek to imitate those who are accomplished in those areas. It might be an athlete, musician, dancer, actor or someone in another discipline we admire and seek to imitate. I remember as a kid choreographing fight scenes with my friends based on what we saw in the movies or on television. We had no real idea what we were doing, but to us, our mimicry looked like those we admired.

At some point we may perceive our own limitations and seek out instruction from a qualified teacher. Finding a good teacher isn't always easy and could be the subject of an entire article. Once a connection is made with a teacher, we find ourselves once again engaged in the act of imitation — this time

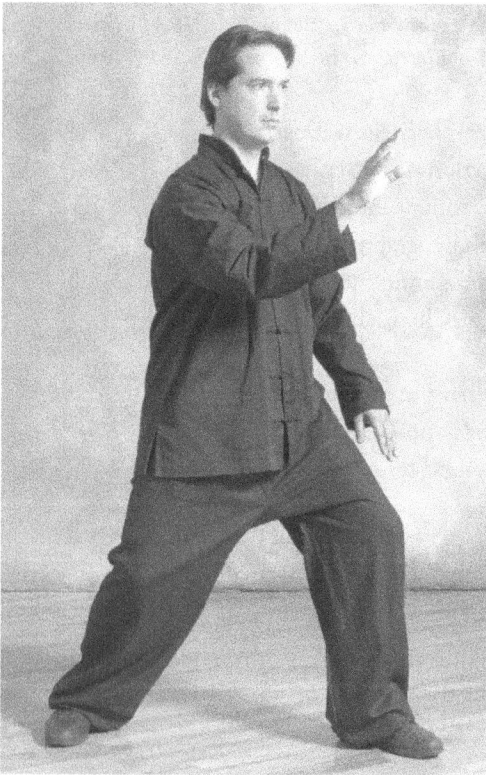

Paul Abdella demonstrates Brush Knee Left.

on a new and deeper level.

As our instruction unfolds, we find that imitating the teacher requires a precision of movement we hadn't formerly encountered. Our new movements contain an understructure of meaning both in principle and execution, which may make our performance of them seem awkward and robotic. Through continued practice and receiving corrections from the teacher, something deeply satisfying begins to occur.

Assimilation: 1. To absorb and incorporate; digest.

In time, the principles behind the movements are understood and assimilated by the mind and body. This process happens incrementally over time and continues on deeper more subtle levels as long as one continues to practice. There is, however, an initial recognition that one's movements have become relaxed and fluid, and they begin to feel like the teacher's movements look. When this occurs, the thin veneer of mere imitation has been transcended and we are on another, more internal, level of practice.

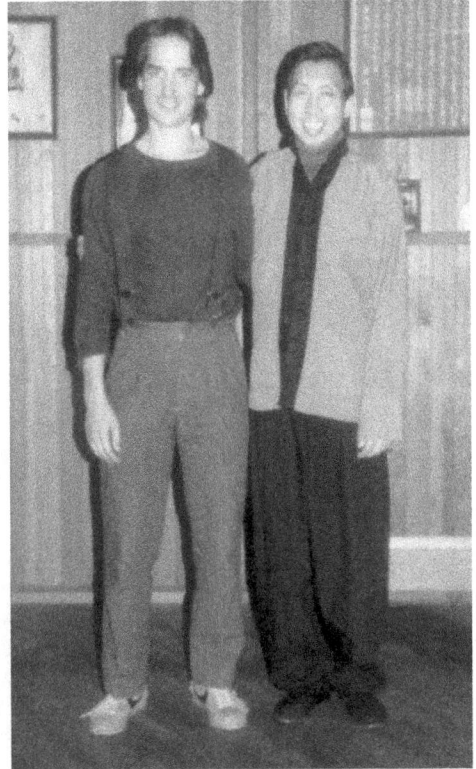

Paul Abdella poses with Master William C.C. Chen at the old Twin Cities T'ai Chi Ch'uan studio in St. Paul, MN, circa 1985.

Over time, as our understanding and assimilation of T'ai-Chi deepens, we begin to naturally personalize our practice. Our areas of interest and specialization become clear, and they shape and guide our T'ai-Chi. We begin to see the principles as flexible guideposts rather than immutable laws. The body begins to follow the dictates of the mind and our natural instinct for creativity begins to emerge. At this point we enter into the stage of innovation.

Innovation: 1. The process of making changes. 2. A new method, custom, idea, etc.

The history of T'ai-Chi is a story of innovation. From its roots in Shaolin through the Chen, Yang, Wu, and other family styles, T'ai-Chi is an art that has passed through the creative minds of many individuals whose willingness to innovate within a tradition has led to its survival and

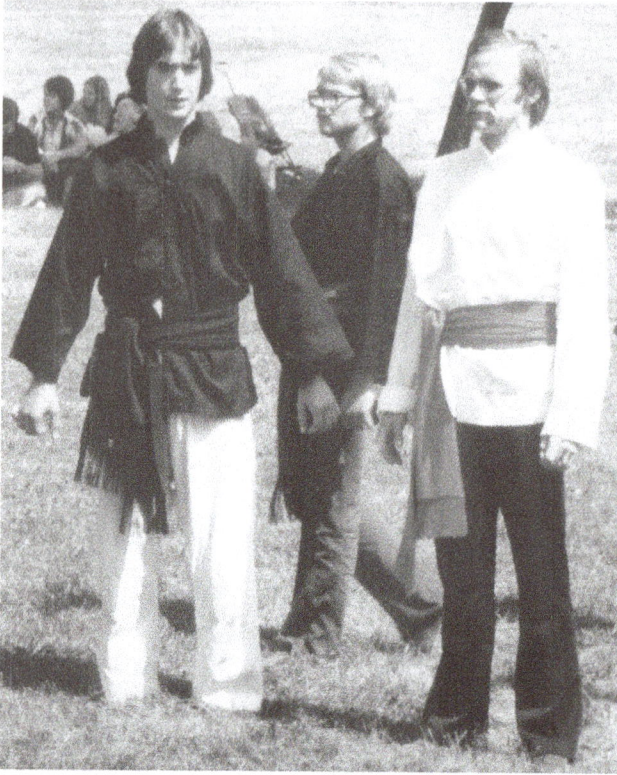

Paul Abdella (left) and his Praying Mantis instructor Doug Anderson (right) at the Camden Summer Festival Demonstration in 1979. The man in the center is unidentified.

continued evolution. Every prominent figure whose innovations have changed the course of the art has passed through the first two stages.

All of us have our own unique reasons for practicing T'ai-Chi, and we each have inherent strengths and weaknesses that influence the way we innovate within our practice. Once all the fundamental principles have been assimilated, someone more oriented toward energy work and meditation would, by necessity, innovate differently than someone more interested in martial arts, for example. Teaching is another vehicle for innovation in T'ai-Chi, since the best teachers have the ability to make the art accessible to diverse groups of people and must remain creative in their approach to teaching.

True innovation, however, is not arbitrary or designed to cover weaknesses in comprehension or technique. Rather, it is a natural outgrowth of having worked slowly and deeply through the first two phases. The first two rules of mastery are, after all: 1. Start at the beginning. And 2. Don't skip any stages.

Cultivating an awareness and enjoyment of the three phases of practice — imitation, assimilation, and innovation — will allow you to continually progress and meet your objectives for as long as you chose to practice.

T'AI-CHI CH'UAN, MEDITATION, AND SELF-CULTIVATION

RAY HAYWARD

Cultivating the self, physically, mentally, emotionally, and spiritually has been the pursuit of Eastern and Western peoples for thousands of years. To be a whole person, the individual worked on perfecting his or her many sides. A guide (teacher, master, or guru) who possessed knowledge, insight, ability, lineage, and accessibility was followed until the student received the full transmission and left to complete the training on his or her own.

Physical cultivation aims at perfecting and mastering the body's functions and abilities. With proper training, the body can be made to be under the control of the mind. Martial arts, healing arts, yoga, and various sports can be used to achieve this goal.

Painting, poetry, calligraphy, and music are just a few of the options for **emotional** cultivation. Through the discipline of classical training methods, emotions can be given avenues of expression and documentation.

Academics, memorization (such as the Confucian training of the memorization of the six ancient books of China), and other scholarly pursuits cultivate the **mental** side.

Spiritual cultivation is realized through meditation, chanting, prayer, and other concentration methods. An ancient esoteric master said, "Those who know themselves, know their lord."

Ray Hayward demonstrates Golden Rooster Standing on One Leg Left.

Through a daily practice of T'ai-Chi Ch'uan and meditation, all aspects of self-cultivation can be exercised. T'ai-Chi provides the physical training such as body movement, two-person practice, and weapon exercises. In T'ai-Chi, the mental aspects are cultivated through memorization of the movements, study of the Classics, and research and reading of instructional material on the art. Master T.T. Liang calls T'ai-Chi the "scholar's martial art" because he feels you have to study as much as you practice.

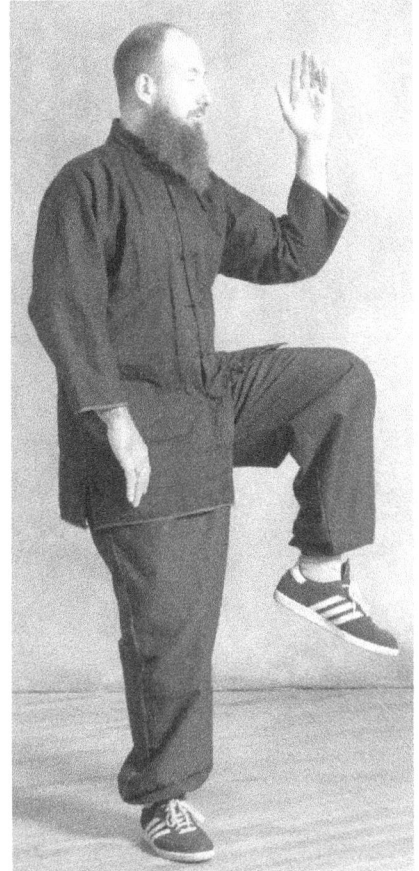

T'ai-Chi embraces all aspects of Taoist meditation. The breathing techniques, energy pathways and points, philosophy, and practice methods train the spiritual side of the individual. Through meditation, individuals can get in touch with and develop their mental, spiritual and emotional selves as well as cultivate their internal energy for good health. Meditation can increase the mental powers of concentration, intuition, and clarity. Mental stress, which is equally as dangerous as physical stress, can be alleviated through a short daily meditation session.

In the past, different groups at the studio emphasized studying weapons, pushing-hands, or researching other styles. My observation of the present group is that, either consciously or not, they are pursuing self-cultivation (which is parallel to my own personal training). With this in mind, I will encourage and help the members to develop a training sequence that fits both their interests and their schedule.

Let me conclude with a quote from my teacher, Shaykh Nazim al-Haqqani: "An individual practice must be like clothing for the practitioner. It is most natural and easy to wear suitable and well-fitting clothing. But if the exercise is too loose, like loose clothes, it will fall off and be left behind by the person. If the practice is too tight, it will restrict the individual and will end up being torn apart. So your practice must fit you correctly to be of use."

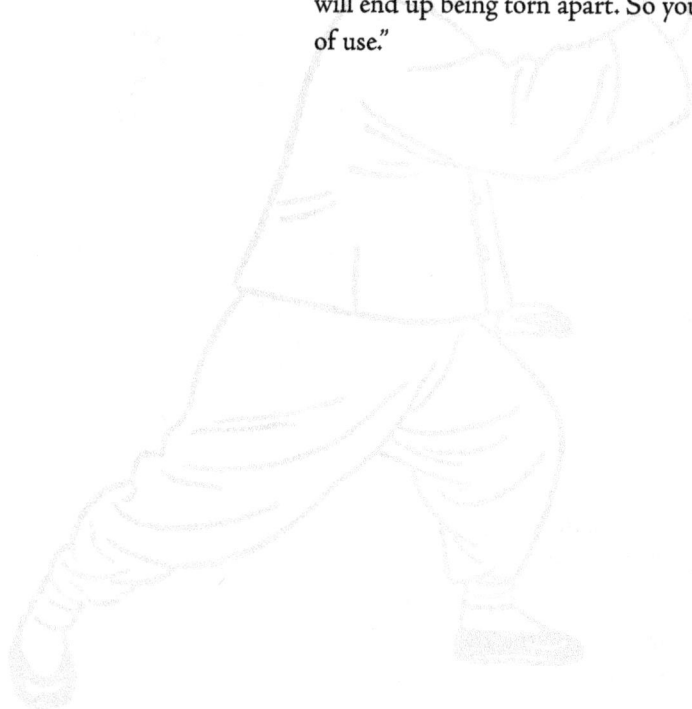

T'ai-Chi Ch'uan, Meditation, and the Five Stimulations

Paul Abdella

The ch'i should be stimulated and the spirit of vitality should be retained internally.

~ *T'ai-Chi Classic*

T'ai-Chi Ch'uan is an art belonging to the internal school of Chinese boxing. This means there is a marriage between the external movement mechanics of the style and the inner qualities of meditation. This article explores T'ai-Chi as moving meditation, and the energy-stimulating properties of the movements themselves.

Meditation

The three essential components of meditation are posture, breath and a quiet mind. In the posture of meditation, the muscles and bones are harmoniously aligned with the force of gravity, thus creating a body that is relaxed and free of tension. As we begin to experience gravity as a source of support rather than a source of tension, the body's energy is naturally stimulated.

Breathing is both a voluntary and an involuntary action. This means that the breath is controlled by two sets of nerves: the voluntary (central) and involuntary (autonomic) nervous systems. Therefore, the breath can act as a bridge between the two and begin to have an influence over what are generally believed to be involuntary processes in the body. When the breath is deep and slow, utilizing the abdomen as well as the chest, more oxygen is drawn into the cells to nourish the body as the nervous system both stimulates the circulation and calms the body down.

When quieting the mind, it is important to learn to control mental activity and the emotions. To do this, the mind is brought to a single focus utilizing a variety of possible techniques such as visualization, sounds, breath-work and the cultivation of emptiness. Any of these techniques can interrupt our emotional patterns and bring our electrical brainwave activity to a lower frequency.

When the three elements of posture, breath and quiet mind are brought together in a practice, the ch'i is stimulated and becomes active. Master T.T. Liang has said, "The ch'i in and of itself is not sufficiently forceful to increase the flow of blood, but if the ch'i is persistently stimulated, it produces heat and becomes powerfully effective in activating the circulation of blood throughout the whole body without any discontinuity. The same principle is illustrated by the conversion of water into steam: the latent invisible power in water is made active enough, effective enough, to drive the pistons of a powerful engine."

THE FIVE STIMULATIONS

The T'ai-Chi Classics state, "In resting, be as still as a mountain peak; in moving, act like the current of a great river."

When T'ai-Chi postures are held, the three essential elements of posture, breath and quiet mind combine together to stimulate the ch'i as if igniting a piece of charcoal. Such is the power of stillness. In moving from posture to posture, the energy is further activated and circulated as if fanning or blowing on the hot coal. This increase in the flow of energy takes place primarily because of five basic actions or stimulations inherent in the movements themselves. These actions are:

+ Expand and contract

+ Rise and sink

+ Full and empty

+ Turn and twist

+ Fast and slow

A closer examination of each action will reveal the hidden power of the T'ai-Chi movements to increase the flow of energy in the body for health and self-defense.

Expand and Contract

From the smallest atom to the far reaches of space, expand and contract is the fundamental rhythm of the universe. When we examine the movements of the Solo Form, we can see the manifestation of this rhythm within each individual posture and from posture to posture within the entire sequence. For example, the postures Single Whip, Lift Hands, and Shoulder Stroke illustrate this idea well. From beginning to end, the posture Single Whip is a series of expanding and contracting gestures, as are Lift Hands and Shoulder Stroke. The finished position of Single Whip looks and feels more expanded than Lift Hands, which looks and feels more expanded than Shoulder Stroke, and so on.

To experience the stimulating power of expand and contract, select a posture from the form and perform it repeatedly with or without footwork as if doing Ch'i-Kung. Soon you will notice that the movement and breath combine together in this rhythm of opposites to stimulate and mobilize your energy.

Rise and Sink

There is a general principle in T'ai-Chi practice that states that the form movements should remain at an even height throughout the sequence (with the exception of the stand-up and squat-down postures). Although this principle is designed to keep a practitioner from arbitrarily bobbing up and down, there are numerous places throughout the form where subtle rise and sink actions stimulate energy and enhance the practical use of a posture.

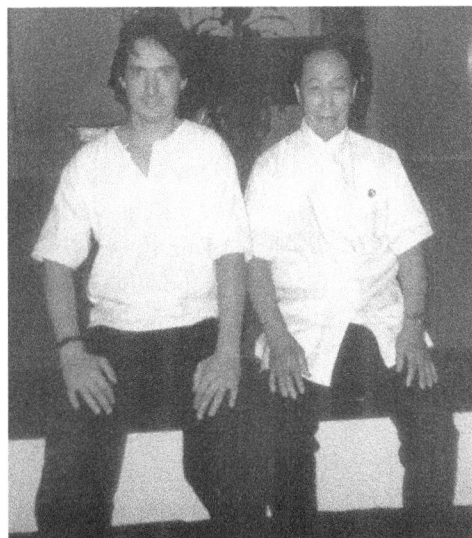

Paul Abdella and Master Wang Yen-nien (one of Master T.T. Liang's teachers) in Washington, D.C. in 1993.

In most postures that finish with the forward hand and forward foot opposite each other, such as Brush Knee, a subtle rising action occurs at the end of a posture caused by the straightening of the rear leg and a slight opening of the chest. In most postures that finish with the forward hand and forward foot on the same side, such as Ward Off, a subtle sinking action occurs at the end of the posture caused by bending the knees slightly and relaxing the chest.

In postures that stand up, such as White Crane Spreads its Wings, the legs are straightened, the chest is opened and the spine is lengthened. In postures that squat down, such as Needle at Sea Bottom, the legs are bent deeply, the chest is relaxed and the back is rounded, then the body rises up again into Fan through the Back.

In all of these examples, the rise and sink actions correspond to the posture applications and also stimulate the movement of cerebrospinal fluid along the spine. Most postures utilize the actions of rise and sink; those that do not are governed by one or more of the other stimulations.

Select a posture with an obvious rise and sink component, such as White Crane Spreads Its Wings, and perform it repeatedly left and right. Soon, the movement of energy along the spine and elsewhere will begin to flow.

Full and Empty

In T'ai-Chi practice, when stepping to advance, retreat, turn left or right, the weight must be shifted from one leg to the other in a gradual and deliberate manner. When the stepping foot is lifted and placed in position, it is in a state of emptiness, leaving the leg that bears the weight completely full. As the weight is slowly shifted from one leg to the other, the status of full and empty in each leg is reversed.

This interchange is continuous throughout the form and applies a steady on/off pressure to the bubbling well points on the soles of the feet — one of the most significant energy centers of the body. In addition, there is a full and empty aspect to the movement of the arms as well as the breath. Together, they unite and stimulate the circulation of energy in the body.

Select a posture from the form such as Push and perform it continuously, paying special attention to the full and empty aspects in the feet, legs, arms and breath.

Turn and Twist

In T'ai-Chi, it is the waist and legs that direct the movement of the postures. There is, however, some confusion as to what is meant by the waist. The pelvis consists of the bones of the hip and sacrum. The lowest section of the spine, the lumbar, is attached to it. Unlike the middle (thoracic) and upper (cervical) sections of the spine, which can bend and rotate in all directions, the lumbar vertebrae cannot rotate or twist very much. Therefore, when the pelvis turns, so do the lumbar vertebrae. This unified movement of the pelvis and lumbar make up what is referred to as the waist in T'ai-Chi.

A common principle in T'ai-Chi is to move the body as a unified whole. When the waist directs the movements in turning side to side, this unity is preserved and the spine is gently stretched and massaged. A small amount of rotation or twist beyond the movement of the waist is acceptable, even beneficial to the spine and nervous system. If the twist comes before the turn (in other words, if the shoulders and chest, not the waist, direct the movements), the movements become segmented, the breath becomes shallow, and the benefits for health and self-defense are diminished.

Select a posture from the form such as Cloud Hands and perform it repeatedly, letting the waist-turn guide the movement. As the waist reaches the limit of the turn and a subtle twist of the upper body moves a little past that point, the stimulation of turn and twist will become apparent.

Fast and Slow

Training forms at different speeds is a traditional and beneficial practice. Slow-speed training in T'ai-Chi develops ch'i by allowing the practitioner to observe, correct and control those elements that interfere with the essentials of meditation and the five stimulations. Training at faster speeds allows one to express that energy for martial purposes.

When practicing T'ai-Chi slowly, there will occur natural shifts in tempo in individual postures and various sections of the form. These subtle shifts in rhythm have a stimulating effect on the body, providing they follow the general principles of the Classics.

Practice a posture, a section of the form, or an entire round of the form at a slow, medium, and fast pace and note the different feeling each produces.

In Conclusion

When the essential elements of meditation — posture, breath, and a quiet mind — are integrated in T'ai-Chi practice, and the movement of the five stimulations fully realized, the body's energy will be full and flowing and ready to obey the dictates of the mind. As Master Liang said, "When the mind mobilizes the intention, and the intention mobilizes the ch'i, and when the ch'i mobilizes the body (circulates throughout the entire body), then the energy of stimulation, which is latent within, will be created. When the mind and ch'i are joined and linked together with the variations of substantial and insubstantial, the energy becomes so very strong and fast that it is like a howling typhoon and fearful waves, or passing clouds and flowing waters, or a flying hawk and a leaping fish, or a hopping rabbit and a swooping falcon, now sinking, now rising, suddenly appearing and suddenly disappearing. The stimulation of the natural greatness of the ch'i is inscrutable like the winds and clouds."

THE THREE ESSENTIALS OF QIGONG

Paul Abdella

Qigong is a system of mind-body exercise designed to revitalize health through breathing, movement, visualization, structural alignment and other natural methods.

Qigong literally means bio-energy (qi) work (gong) or, working with the energy of life. The Chinese have practiced Qigong for thousands of years and now it is becoming popular in the West, as its health-giving properties become better known. Although the methods of Qigong are numerous and varied, there are some common principles they all share. The three essential elements included in all Qigong practices are: 1. Posture, 2. Breath, and 3. A quiet mind.

This article will introduce each element separately, detailing some of the physiology and function of each while relating them to the whole of Qigong as a general practice. Whether you are already practicing Qigong or just starting out, having a deeper understanding of these essential building blocks will enhance your practice.

PART ONE: POSTURE

When the lowest vertebrae are plumb and erect, the spirit of vitality reaches to the top of the head. When the top of the head is held as if suspended from above, the whole body feels light and agile.
~ *T'ai-Chi Classic*

Posture refers to the effect of gravity on the alignment of bones and muscles. With the spine as the central pillar of the body's structure, its relationship to the head and pelvis should be the primary focus for developing the proper posture for Qigong practice. Any disharmony to this alignment results in a diminished flow of energy to the body. Energy blockages in the body ultimately result in illness.

The spine is a beautiful example of functional design. The bones, discs, and ligaments make up the spinal column and are arranged in four natural flowing curves. Together they maintain the structure of the trunk, allow for mobility, and act as a shock absorber.

Most importantly perhaps, the spine houses and protects the spinal cord, the branch of the central nervous system extending from the brain down through the trunk of the body. The spinal cord provides energy and control of the body by making the muscles work. The autonomic nervous system also descends along the spine and is responsible for organ and glandular function, among other things.

Over time, poor posture, incorrect body mechanics, stress, and the general loss of strength and flexibility can erode the structure of the spinal column and diminish the full functioning of the nervous system. It is important that we correct and maintain proper alignment in all our activities so as to circulate energy freely and cultivate our health.

Gravity

The effect of gravity on the spine is to compress the discs that lie between the vertebrae. If the spine is aligned properly during your daily activities, the discs will naturally decompress during sleep time, making you as much as half an inch taller when you rise the next morning. Astronauts who experience zero gravity in space for extended periods can come back to Earth as much as two inches taller.

If your daily routine demands long periods of time in unnatural and stressful positions, such as hunching over a computer terminal or doing repetitive tasks with poor body mechanics, your muscles will develop tension patterns that misalign the spine and may not release during sleep. This creates a continual state of compression in the spine, which has a detrimental effect to the circulation of energy, and to the structure itself.

When the body is aligned with the force of gravity, it naturally feels relaxed, breathing becomes deep and unrestricted, and the mind becomes more aware of tense or blocked areas of the body. Ultimately, the goal is for the spine to be held upright, as if suspended from the crown of the head by a string that gently pulls upward, while the base of the spine is pulled down by slightly tucking the pelvis. If this is maintained, a feeling of openness and release is created in the torso and neck.

Standing

Although an open and vertical spine is essential to good posture, the position of the feet, knees, hips, chest, elbows and shoulders in relation to it is also extremely important. The following is a description of a Qigong standing practice, including how each of the elements are integrated.

Stand with the feet shoulder-width and parallel. Keep the feet flat on the floor and shift the weight forward onto the balls of the feet, then back to the heels; repeat a few times. Then settle the weight in between, where you feel equal pressure on the balls and heels. Relax into this position as if the feet were deflating balloons.

Straighten the legs without locking the knees. This is called standing with soft knees. Feel this push the head upward, lengthening the spine as if the head were suspended and being pulled from above. Although the spine straightens, it is not rigid like a pole, but rather, flexible like a piece of elastic. Imagine the elastic has beads along its length representing the vertebrae, and as the elastic is elongated, space opens between the beads.

Gently tuck the hips under, which pulls the elastic spine downward. It is important not to tuck the hips too much, as is common by many Qigong and T'ai-Chi practitioners — this can be stressful to the lower back. Personal comfort level should dictate the degree of tuck. Relax the abdomen (no one's looking!), relax the chest, allowing it to be neither collapsed, nor extended. Lift the shoulders as if shrugging then let them drop. Tension is commonly held in this area, so let the shoulders sink low and let the arms hang freely.

The relationship between the elbows and shoulders is important. When the elbow rises, so will the shoulder. Often this builds tension in the shoulders and neck with prolonged activity. While performing work with the arms, observe the position of the elbows and strive to lower them as much as possible. This will, to a large degree, eliminate the buildup of tension in this area.

Let the head feel centered and balanced on the neck, not straining forward like a horse trying to win a race. If the head is forward, place one finger on the space between the upper lip and nose and push the head back to its natural place on top of the spine.

Now, take a few moments and stand in this position bringing, your awareness to your

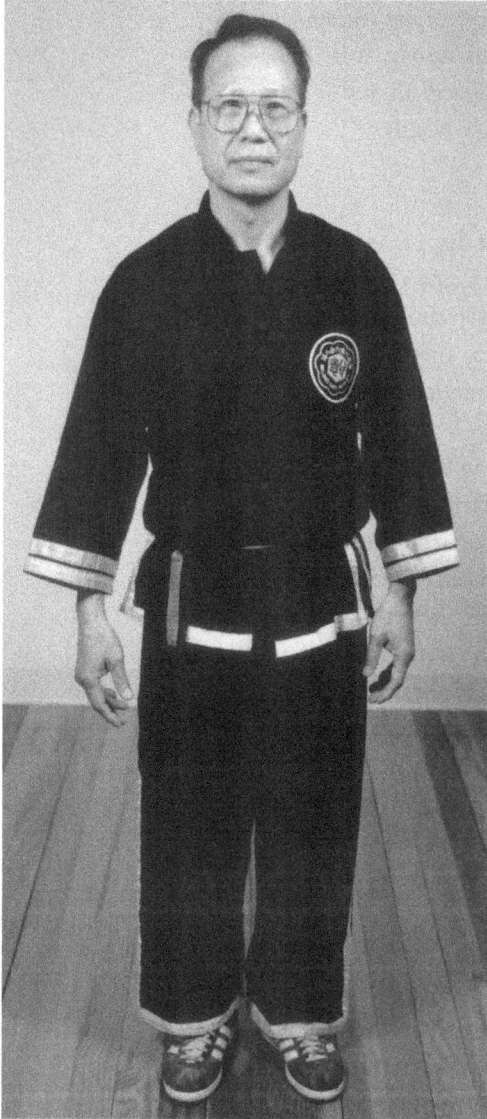

Grandmaster Wai-lun Choi demonstrates the first I-Ch'uan standing meditation posture, sometimes called "Wu-Ji" or "the Limitless."

alignment. Feel the body deeply relax as you stand in this natural posture. You will become aware of areas of tension and misalignment as you maintain this new position. Allow the body to adjust.

Relaxation

Next, just as you created your Qigong posture one piece at a time from the ground up, imagine a wave of relaxation traveling downward from head to toe. This wave of relaxation can be compared to drawing a tea bag up out of the water. As the tea bag is drawn upward by the string and suspended from above, the liquid within it is slowly drained from top to bottom until finally the last few drops are released from below.

Proceed from head to toe: feel the face and neck relax, the shoulders lower and relax, chest and upper back, arms, abdomen and lower back, hips, legs. Feel all the joints open and clear, then let it all release through the feet into the ground.

Again, stand for a few moments, bringing your awareness inward, then repeat the sequence for creating alignment from bottom to top: feet flat, legs straightened, spine lengthened, knees soft, hips tucked, abdomen and chest relaxed, shoulders down, arms relaxed, head centered, eyes softly focused. Then repeat the downward relaxation, allowing the cycle to continue as long as you can comfortably stand.

This is a simple but powerful Qigong practice, which not only builds proper alignment but also deepens the breath and quiets the mind. As you do standing practice, you will become aware of areas of tension, emotions, misalignments and other conditions that may require additional relief to help correct your posture. Remedies could include stretching, massage, structural work, and other healing modalities. In time and with constant practice, the body will be realigned and the power of posture will reveal itself in the creation of radiant health.

PART TWO: BREATH

One must breathe the essence of life, regulate one's respiration to preserve one's spirit and keep the body relaxed.
~ *The Yellow Emperor's Classic of Internal Medicine*

Breath is the primary source of energy in the body — the essence of life itself. It is therefore a natural object of meditation and is used in

Qigong to form a link between the body and mind and to increase the available energy in the body. To find out how the breath is used to accomplish this let's examine some of the physical, mental, emotional and spiritual qualities of breathing.

Physical Breath

The physical body is comprised of millions of tiny individual living units called cells. The life of the body is dependent upon a continuous source of energy to the cells, which is provided when oxygen combines with nutrient fuel derived from our food and is burned within the cell to release energy.

This process could be compared to an automobile engine where fuel and air are mixed and exploded in what is the equivalent of our cells — the combustion chamber or cylinder. This explosion releases energy, which is used to turn the wheels of the car. Unlike the combustion chamber of an automobile engine where fuel is burned rapidly to create an explosion of energy, the fuel in our cells is burned very slowly over time, producing energy at a slow, steady rate.

When something is burned, a natural waste product is produced, such as the carbon ash remaining after a campfire has burned out. Carbon dioxide is the waste product produced when fuel is burned in our cells. It must be removed if the cells are to remain healthy. This is the function of the exhalation phase of breathing, while the inhalation phase draws oxygen from the air we breathe into the body and delivers it to the cells. This continuous gaseous exchange insures that the body receives the energy it needs.

Finding a way to draw the maximum amount of oxygen into the body with the minimum amount of effort is essential to the practice of Qigong. By looking at the mechanics of breathing, we can understand how best to achieve this in our practice.

The physical act of breathing occurs in the torso of the body. If we imagine the torso as a cylinder, we can divide it into two simple sections: the chest, which houses the heart and lungs, and the abdomen, which contains the organs of digestion and elimination. The diaphragm, a thin sheet of muscle that attaches to the lower ribs, sternum and spinal column, divides the two sections. In its resting position, the diaphragm is not flat; it billows up into the chest cavity like a dome or parachute. This is its position during exhalation.

The diaphragm, like any muscle when it contracts, will shorten and take up the smallest surface area possible, which flattens the dome shape and increases the space in the chest cavity. Because the lungs are covered with a very thin double layer of tissue that is attached to the inner surface of the chest wall and the topside of the diaphragm, any movement of the chest or diaphragm will be transmitted to the lungs. Thus, if the chest expands out or the diaphragm moves down, the lungs will be expanded, creating suction and causing air to flow into them.

These are the two primary ways air moves into the lungs. They are called chest breathing and diaphragmatic breathing, respectively. It is diaphragmatic breathing, sometimes known as abdominal or natural breathing that is generally used in the practice of Qigong. It is physiologically the most efficient way of breathing, since most of the blood in the lungs moves with the force of gravity to the lower portions, and it is there that the greatest expansion occurs when the diaphragm is lowered.

Chest breathing is not as efficient in bringing air to this portion of the lungs, so less oxygen is mixed with the blood. More energy is required to expand and contract the ribs to achieve the same blood/oxygen mix as deep abdominal breathing, which results in the need to take more frequent breaths.

Due to the extra energy expended, more blood needs to circulate through the lungs, which, in turn, increases the workload on the heart. If the oxygen requirements of the body are great, such as in athletic performance, a combination of diaphragmatic and chest breathing can be used. Because chest breathing is efficient in bringing air to the middle and upper portions of the lungs, starting a breath in the abdomen and letting the expansion smoothly flow up into the chest will distribute a greater volume of air throughout the lungs: creating a complete breath.

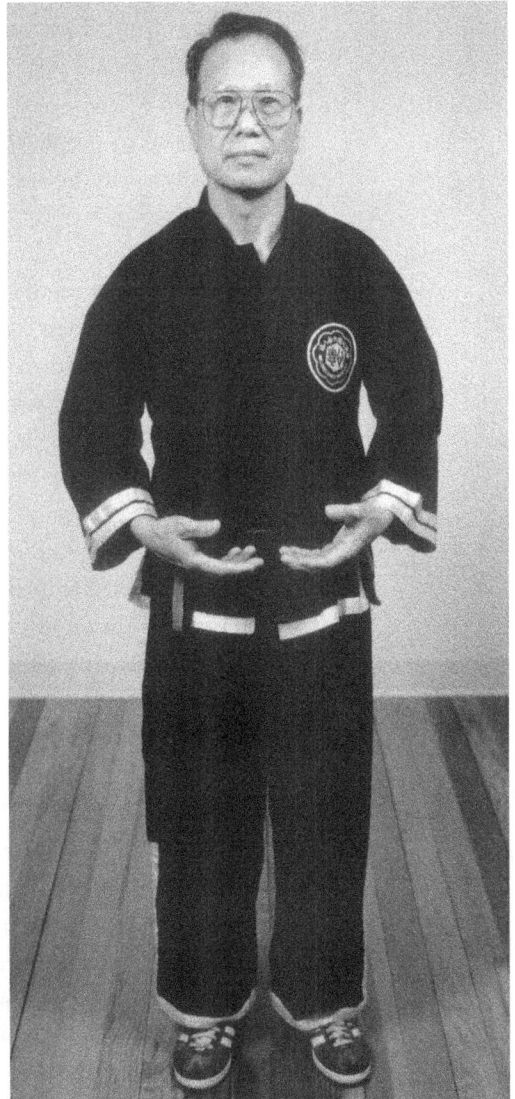

Grandmaster Wai-lun Choi demonstrates the second I-Ch'uan standing meditation posture, sometimes called "Chuc-San" or "Packaged and Wrapped Up."

We all began life as abdominal breathers (infants and small children must breathe this way until the bony structure of the chest matures), but if it has been a while since you were regularly breathing in this manner, a quick "how to" review might help you get started again.

Get comfortable in a reclining position face up on a flat surface such as a bed, sofa or carpeted floor (a small neck pillow is okay to use). Place one hand on your chest and the other on your abdomen. Take a moment or two and observe your breath. Try and feel with the hands where your breath is located — is it in the chest, abdomen or both, perhaps? It is important to simply observe the breath and not to force the breathing in any way. Then move the hand that is on the chest to the abdomen, so that both hands are resting there.

Gradually begin to expand the abdomen using the abdominal muscles as you inhale. Feel the abdomen expand and draw air in like a bellows. Relax the abdomen completely to exhale. Continue this sequence for a while until the breath becomes relaxed, smooth, and rhythmic.

In the resting position, the body's energy requirements are slight, so a large expansion of the abdomen is unnecessary. In time, as the body relearns how to breathe diaphragmatically, you can experiment with expanding more and taking in larger volumes of air.

Practice this reclining breathing exercise daily, eventually not using the hands, until it becomes relaxed and natural. Then begin practicing in a standing position until this too becomes relaxed and natural. Eventually, let diaphragmatic breathing replace chest breathing as your normal breathing pattern and watch as your stress and tension levels diminish while your energy levels increase.

Mental/Emotional Breath

Breathing can be performed consciously as well as unconsciously because breathing is controlled by two sets of nerves: the voluntary (central) nervous system and the involuntary (autonomic) nervous system. The breath acts as a bridge between these two systems. To illustrate this concept, try holding your breath — this is a conscious act performed by the voluntary nervous system. As you will soon discover, if a threat to your survival is perceived by the involuntary nervous system, it overrides the voluntary one and you are forced to resume breathing.

The voluntary or central nervous system controls our motor skills such as muscle function, sensory and emotional awareness, speech and other functions associated with the brain. The involuntary or autonomic nervous system regulates the function of our vital organs and glands. These vital organs (heart, lungs, liver, kidneys, etc.) are not normally considered to be under our voluntary control. However, we know the breath can operate voluntarily, and therefore we can begin to regulate the movement of the lungs through deep controlled breathing. The lungs and heart work together, and as the lungs begin to work more efficiently the heart is regulated and also works more efficiently.

The involuntary nervous system has two branches that work in harmonious opposition to each other — one that stimulates and accelerates the function of the vital organs (sympathetic system) and the other that slows down the functions of the organs (parasympathetic system). A healthy balance and general tone of this involuntary nervous system is critical to the health of the organs and body.

When the balance and tone of this system is off, it can produce irregular heart rhythms, high blood pressure, poor circulation, digestive disorders and other illness, since these are all controlled by this set of nerves. By working with the breath during Qigong, you can influence and tone the autonomic nervous system and affect many of the involuntary functions in the body for the betterment of your health.

In addition to affecting the autonomic nervous system, breathing has a direct connection and influence on our emotional states. Recall an incident where you were angry or afraid and you will probably recall breathing that was rapid, shallow and irregular. The emotions' effect on the breath is coordinated by the autonomic nervous system.

If the emotions can affect breathing, breathing can in turn affect the emotions. You cannot be in a rage if your breathing is slow, deep, smooth and quiet. It is not always possible to control the external conditions that affect our emotions, but you can use your breath to influence the part of your nervous system that slows down organ function, bringing you to a more calm and centered place from which to make decisions and take actions. Regular Qigong exercises will cultivate the breath control needed to influence our emotions in a more positive way.

Spirit Breath

The words for spirit and breath are the same in many languages. In Chinese, *Qi (chee)*; Japanese, *Ki*; Sanskrit, *Prana*; Greek, *Pneuma*; and Latin, *Spiritus*. The common understanding these ancient cultures had for breath stems from their observation and experience of the cycles of life.

All of life pulsates to the universal rhythm of expansion and contraction and the duality of opposites that cannot be separated. From day and night, growth and decay, to the beat and pause of the human heart — from the positive and negative charge of the smallest atom to the expansion of the universe (which science tells us will one day contract again, completing one cosmic breath) — this rhythm truly manifests in all things.

Einstein said that "matter is energy" and energy cannot be destroyed, it can only be transformed. Spirit is the animating vital force in all-living things, and the breath represents the movement of spirit in matter. To cultivate the breath is to cultivate the spirit.

Part Three: Quiet Mind

When the mind is at peace, the world too is at peace.
~ *Layman P'ang*

For most of our waking day, our minds are focused on the external world. From the distractions of current events to the demands of our careers, the mind exists in a world "out there" rather than "in here." When we do bring the mind inside, often it is to relive a memory (the past) or indulge a fantasy (the future), and we miss the space and time where life is truly lived: the present moment. This tendency to flee the present makes learning to calm and quiet the mind and bring it into focus an essential element in the practice of Qigong.

The Mind's Influence on the Body

The Chinese have likened the mind to a wild horse running unbridled in any direction it chooses, or a monkey swinging from tree to tree. Left untamed, its boundless energy is

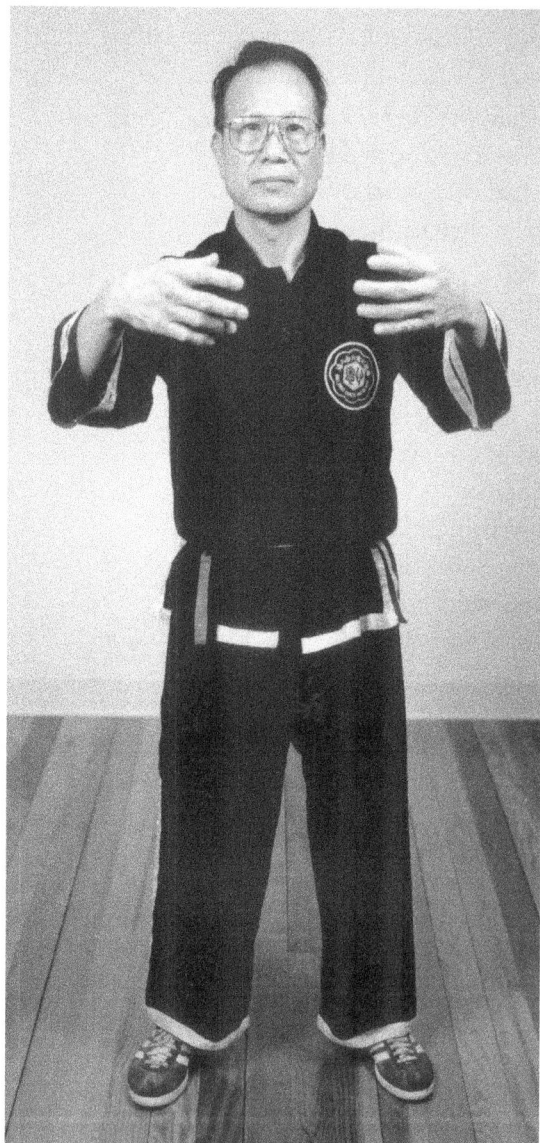

Grandmaster Wai-lun Choi demonstrates the third I-Ch'uan standing meditation posture, commonly called "Embrace the Moon."

never harnessed for any fruitful purpose. Thoughts appear and disappear like passing clouds with little awareness of their deeper effect on the body, mind, and spirit.

Most of us can recall an incident in our lives where we felt anger, sadness, joy or some other emotion and instantly feel these emotions return. Indeed, science has recorded changes to body temperature, respiration, heart rate and other biological functions with the memory of a past event.

Let's examine some of the ways in which our thoughts and perceptions create physiological changes in the body. A man we'll call Joe returns home from a long, frustrating day at work. He represented his department in making an important presentation to the president and board of directors of his company. It wasn't well received. The result was a loss of respect for Joe by his superiors and coworkers, a diminished budget for his department and possibly some lost jobs.

In recounting the day's events, he begins to realize that inadequate information and unrealistic deadlines from his supervisor contributed to the failure of the project, as did incompetent support from his coworkers — yet he is being held responsible. As Joe reviews the events in his mind, his disappointment and frustration turn to anger and depression.

If Joe's heart rate, blood pressure and other vital signs were measured during this memory of events, some alarming statistics would appear.

The heart speeds up and slows down in different beat patterns. Scientists measure these beat-to-beat changes in heart rate as heart rate variability (HRV). Almost any stimulus to the brain, such as thoughts and emotions, will influence these heart rate changes. Joe's HRV patterns became erratic and jerky, indicating that his sympathetic and parasympathetic nervous systems are out of sync with each other. These two branches of the nervous system work together to regulate heart rate and blood pressure, as well as to establish communication between the brain and vital organs.

When this system is out of balance, blood vessels constrict, blood pressure rises, breathing becomes shallow and energy is depleted. If this happens consistently, you can become hypertensive, which greatly increases your risk of heart disease and stroke. The brain may also flood the body with the stress hormone cortisol, which effectively shuts the parasympathetic nervous system down. This nervous system imbalance is not only detrimental to the heart, but to the brain, hormonal, and immune systems as well.

In the immune system is an antibody called IgA (immunoglobulin A) that protects us against colds, flu, and infections of the respiratory and urinary tracts. In a study that compared the effects of anger versus compassion on average IgA levels, it was found that one five-minute episode of recalling an experience of anger and frustration caused an immediate but short rise in IgA, followed by a depletion so severe it took the body more than six hours to restore normal production of the antibody. The study showed that recalling a single episode of anger and frustration could depress the immune system for almost an entire day!

The same study showed that one five-minute memory episode of the emotions care and compassion caused an immediate and much larger rise in IgA, followed by a return to normal levels. However, the levels then gradually climbed above the normal level for the next six hours. Other studies have shown that feelings of joy and happiness increase white blood cell counts, further boosting the body's immune system.

There is overwhelming evidence of the degenerative effects that stress and negative emotions have on the body, and increasing evidence showing the regenerative power of positive mental and emotional states. Knowing how to shift into a state of mind that promotes optimum performance of the body's biological functions is necessary if we are to offset the day-to-day stress of modern life. Qigong provides such knowledge.

Entering Tranquility

In order to quiet the mind for Qigong practice, one must bring under control three basic factors: external environment, mental activity and emotional activity.

Environment. When beginning your practice, it is important to be in an environment free of distractions. The space should be free of unpleasant odors, lighting, colors, objects, and noise. The environment should be aesthetically pleasing and engaging to as many of the senses as possible. For example, use incense or fresh air from an open window to engage the sense of smell. Soft, subdued lighting or natural light, muted, harmonious colors, an uncluttered room simple in design, sounds from nature or quiet music can all enhance the process of quieting the mind. The ability to control some of the senses at deeper levels is a benefit of regular practice. For example, our sense of hearing has an inner and outer aspect. If an external sound is distracting to us it is possible to focus on our inner hearing in the form of a word, phrase, or other sound to engage the sense in a pleasing way and allow the mind to become quiet and still. In time you will learn to adapt to less than ideal surroundings as your mind develops and becomes undisturbed by external factors.

Mental activity. To reduce mental activity, one must let go of all extraneous thoughts and bring the awareness to a single focus. This puts the mind in a meditative or alpha state where the electrical brainwave patterns have slowed from those of our normal waking state. When this occurs in the mind, the body will follow by activating the parasympathetic nervous system, which slows the heart rate and calms the body down.

Any number of techniques can be introduced to quiet the mind, such as focusing on energy centers and pathways in the body, repeating sounds, words, or phrases (audibly or internally), or holding a thought or visual image in the mind. The most commonly used technique, however, is to bring the awareness to the breath. Breathing is both a voluntary and an involuntary process that allows the meditator some influence over the lungs, heart, and other automatic processes.

Begin your practice by adjusting your posture, calming the breath, and letting go of your thoughts. Then introduce the focus/awareness technique(s). Utilize whatever techniques work best for you or are inherent in the particular Qigong practice you are doing.

Practitioners of Qigong and meditation will generally fit one of two basic categories. They will posses either a yin- or yang-type personality. Yin-type people tend to "zone out" in meditation, making techniques that require concentration and focus better suited to balance this tendency. These might include concentration on specific energy points or vocalizing stimulating sounds. Yang-type people are easily over stimulated by focusing too hard on something and would benefit from cultivating a more general awareness of the body and its release of tension. The breath is a balanced place to center the awareness for both yin and yang personalities. Spend some time with different methods to assess this tendency in yourself if you don't already know.

As you practice, thoughts will reappear and consume your attention. When you notice this occurring, simply let the thoughts go and bring the awareness back to a single focus by reintroducing the breath or other techniques. In time, and with consistent practice, the mind will quickly settle into a tranquil state and remain there for the duration of your practice.

Emotional activity. The mind is essentially a pattern-making computer. It seeks to create patterns of information, store them, and then recognize them. Some patterns are built into the mind and manifest as instinctual behavior. The most important property of the mind, however, is its ability to create its own patterns. The mind doesn't discriminate between an information pattern that is positive and one that's negative, just that it is repeated and stored in the mind/body for immediate or future use. As we've already examined, the emotions can induce powerful physiological changes to the body and mind that can either harm or heal.

Harnessing the power of the emotions is essential if we are to reach deeper levels of tranquility in our practice. When negative emotions overwhelm us, we typically set up a kind of repetitive tape loop that is played over and over in our minds. This is like putting a videotape in the VCR and playing it continuously.

Let's go back and rejoin our friend Joe and his conflict at work. As Joe reviews the events of his difficult day, he begins to create a pattern sequence in his mind that goes something like this: I FAILED. IT WAS MY FAULT. I'M ANGRY. I'M DEPRESSED... I FAILED, etc.

In order to offset the negative impact of this thought pattern Joe must get to a neutral emotional state in order to alter his perceptions of the situation and reprogram a more positive emotional response. In other words, Joe needs to press the pause button on his VCR.

To get to a neutral state, interrupt the thought pattern, and then take a time-out by bringing the awareness to the breath until it is slow, smooth, and deep. Next, bring the awareness to the area around the heart. Imagine you are breathing through the heart.

Keep the mind and breath in this area for a minute or two. Recall a time when you experienced compassion, joy, or some other positive emotion and take some time to re-experience those feelings. Ask the heart sincerely for intuition and guidance in restructuring a response to the current situation, one that will reduce the stress reaction and allow for a new, more balanced perception to emerge.

Although this may seem simplistic, there is a scientific basis for its effectiveness.

The heart is our main power center in the body. Electrically, it is 40 to 60 times more powerful than the brain. This electrical signal can be measured at any point on the body, indicating that power from the heart permeates every cell.

As mentioned earlier, the balance between the sympathetic and parasympathetic nervous systems establishes two-way communication between the brain and heart and other internal organs. There is a third nerve pathway called the baroreceptor system that originates in the heart and sends communications to the brain. When stimulated, it sends information to the higher brain centers, where perception and learning activate this pathway.

Your perceptions trigger mental and emotional activity, which stimulates the nervous system. This electrical stimulation in turn affects heart rate, blood pressure, hormonal production and immune response, which combine to create a healthy body and mind. Balancing mental and emotional activity through the practice of quieting the mind insures that these communication links in the body operate at their highest level.

In learning to practice Qigong, we must integrate the three essentials of posture, breath, and quiet mind in a natural and gradual manner. With consistent practice, we will develop control of the conscious mind, influence the involuntary systems and remain in a state of awareness that allows us to cultivate wisdom and reach our highest potential.

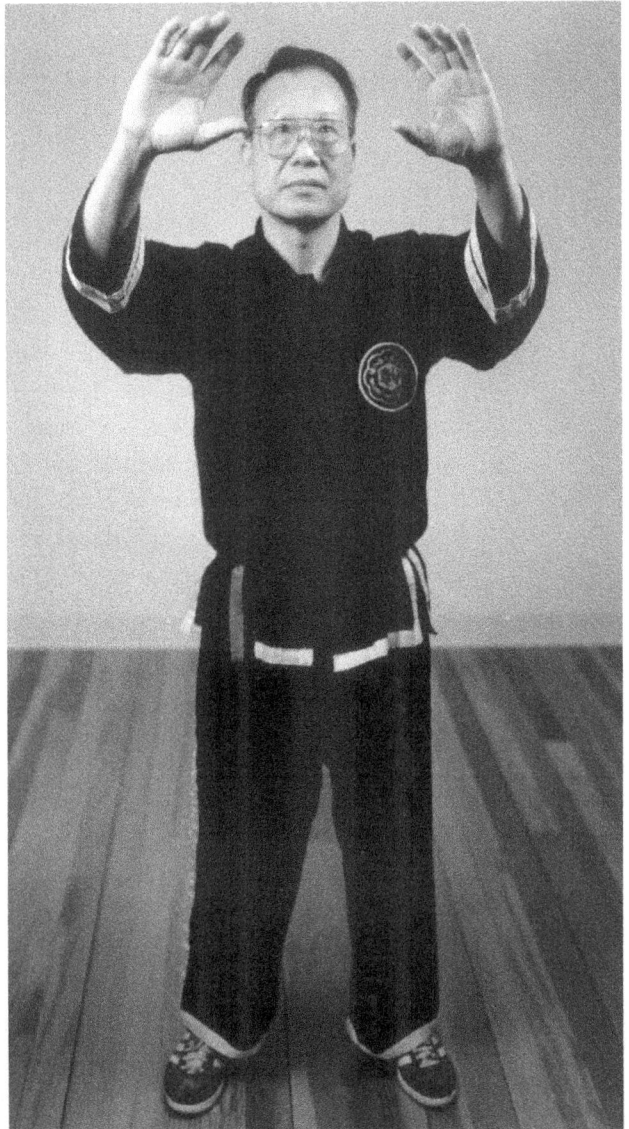

Grandmaster Wai-lun Choi demonstrates the fourth I-Ch'uan standing meditation posture, sometimes called "Two Hands Support Heaven." A strong spirit of vitality can be seen emanating from his eyes.

The What, Why, When and How of Pushing-Hands

Ray Hayward

In this article, I will explain real pushing-hands techniques, practices, theories, and some benefits you can gain from this essential T'ai-Chi practice.

Over the years, instructors from other schools have come wanting to learn pushing-hands or take their knowledge further. They have read about soft and yielding, but once they leave the most fundamental of practices, they become, as Master Liang says, "two bulls fighting." This is a lesson for students as well as teachers.

We may read many books about T'ai-Chi theory and pushing-hands, and we may grasp the ideas, but it takes a good teacher with the correct method and a certain degree of skill of his or her own to guide us through the pitfalls of tension, ego and competition. We are fortunate that our teacher, Master T.T. Liang, is an expert in this field.

What is Pushing-Hands?

The first question is "What is pushing-hands?" Pushing-hands, otherwise known as push-hands, sensing-hands, outreaching-hands, joint-hands, sticking-hands, or *tui-shou* (which means a hand that reaches out by sense of touch, i.e. pushing), is a practice involving two partners using any one of five categories of methods, for the basic purpose of self-knowledge. Lao-Tse says in the *Tao Te Ch'ing*, "To know others is knowledge, to know yourself is enlightenment."

These practices involve fixed and active steps, prearranged sequences, "feeding" sequences (which literally means I will give you certain techniques over and over again), and many ways in between, leading up to free-style, which is totally spontaneous, improvised, and the summation of all partner training. The way we gain this knowledge is by working toward yin goals and yang goals, which I explain later in this article.

Pushing-Hands Drills

The first category of practice is the pushing-hands drills. The drills involve two partners taking turns between active and passive, offense and defense, issuing energy and neutralizing energy. Besides laying a foundation for more complicated practices, the drills help you to focus on a particular attack and a particular defense (which I like to call "problem" and "solution"). The drills illustrate the defenses for pushes, pulls, strikes and ch'in-na. They emphasize that the yielding, defensive aspect is accompanied by shifting back, while the attacking, issuing energy is accompanied by shifting forward. Leading, following, and many aspects of the philosophy of yin and yang are easily understood and experienced in the drills. Also in the drills is a set of basic sticking hands, which is mainly striking attacks and their appropriate defenses.

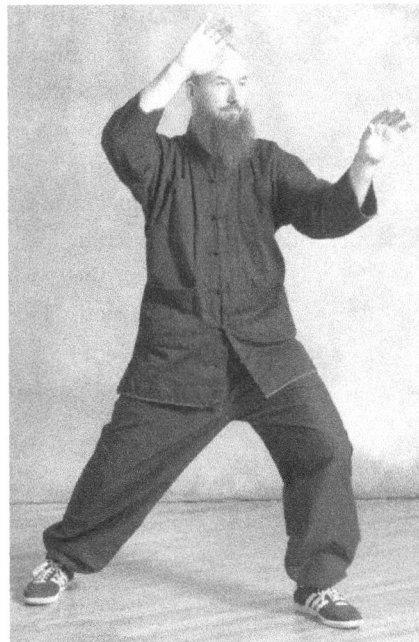

Ray Hayward demonstrates Fan Through the Back.

Pushing-Hands Methods

The next category we call the methods. This is what other schools think of when they want to do pushing-hands but, as you'll see, this is a higher level. The methods are either one- or two-handed, with vertical and horizontal circles, using the four directions (the postures of Ward Off, Roll Back, Press and Push) alternating back and forth in offensive and defensive patterns. The methods are also practiced fixed-step, which means you stay in place, and active-step, which means you can move around. When we progress from the drills to the methods, we start to combine and use multiple techniques.

Ta-Lu

Another category is called Ta-Lu, which literally means "big Roll Back." Ta-Lu uses the four corner techniques, which are pull, split, elbow and shoulder, and the five steps, which are advance, retreat, left, right, and central equilibrium. In Ta-Lu, the techniques are generally bigger; therefore the attacks and defenses need footwork to support them.

As a package, the four directions of pushing-hands and the four corners of Ta-Lu are what we call the eight energies, which are eight ways we may attack our partner's centerline or balance (this subject will be dealt with in the how-to part of this article). The eight energies combined with the five steps are commonly called the 13 postures, and they make up all the variations in T'ai-Chi, whether it's solo, two-person or with weapons.

San-Shou

The final category is called San-Shou, which translates as "free-hand" and is also called freestyle. The T'ai-Chi two-person form is called San-Shou because it freely mixes and combines techniques from the Solo Form, the drills, the methods, and the Ta-Lus in a choreographed sequence to teach you how to deal with all kinds of attacks. Kicking, punching, pushing, pulling, locking of joints, sweeping, knock-downs, and other various problems are dealt with using relaxed T'ai-Chi solutions. The concepts of *hua* (neutralize), *na* (control), and *da* (strike), are clearly shown in each and every technique.

The two-person form teaches many concepts and strategies for sparring and self-defense (for example, how to protect your territory while attacking your partner's territory, or how to apply the classic, "You must gain a good opportunity and a superior position").

Besides the basic sequence, there are many ways to practice and alter the two-person form, which is the jump-off stage for true freestyle practice. After mastering the two-person form in all its variations, you will be ready for true freestyle in the way the old masters practiced it.

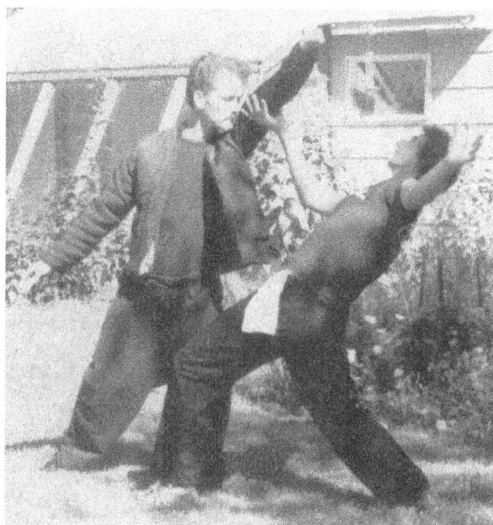
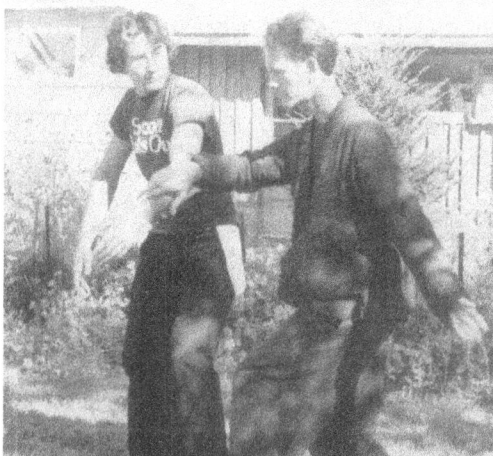

Ray Hayward and Paul Gallagher practicing San-Shou at Wu-Ming Valley House in Amherst, Massachusetts in 1981.

Pushing—Hands Goals

Once you know what you are going to practice, one thing that seems to get confusing is the goal for practice. I call these yin and yang goals.

Yin goals

+ Test partner's relaxation and sinking

+ Use a push or pull to unbalance partner

+ Make partner take one step back

+ Make partner take two steps back

- Uproot partner (both feet leave the ground simultaneously)

- Push partner back past a line

- Push partner into a mattress on the wall

- Maneuver partner out of a circle

- Touch partner's body or trunk (which is the foundation for sticking-hands)

Yang goals

- Partner touches one hand to the floor for balance

- Partner touches two hands to the floor to regain balance

- Body/trunk touches the ground from a push, pull, knock-down, throw or sweep

- Lock partner's joint with ch'in-na

- Strike partner with any possible body part (hand, elbow, head, foot, etc.)

In short, yin goals are for sensitivity, health, non-violence, and non-martial arts gains, while yang goals are more aggressive and dangerous, and are for self-defense and fighting. Great care must be taken to protect practitioners from serious injury.

Why Practice Pushing-Hands?

Why should we practice pushing-hands? Isn't the Solo Form enough? Can I substitute weapons or ch'i-kung? If I'm not interested in self-defense, why should I do pushing-hands? What will I get from all this? Let's see if we can answer these questions and clear up any misconceptions.

T'ai-Chi can be divided into four categories: health, self-defense, philosophy and meditation. We could say that these categories are like four benefits, uses, or even ways to look at the art, although they exist together at all times.

Let's use each of these categories to see the benefits of pushing-hands.

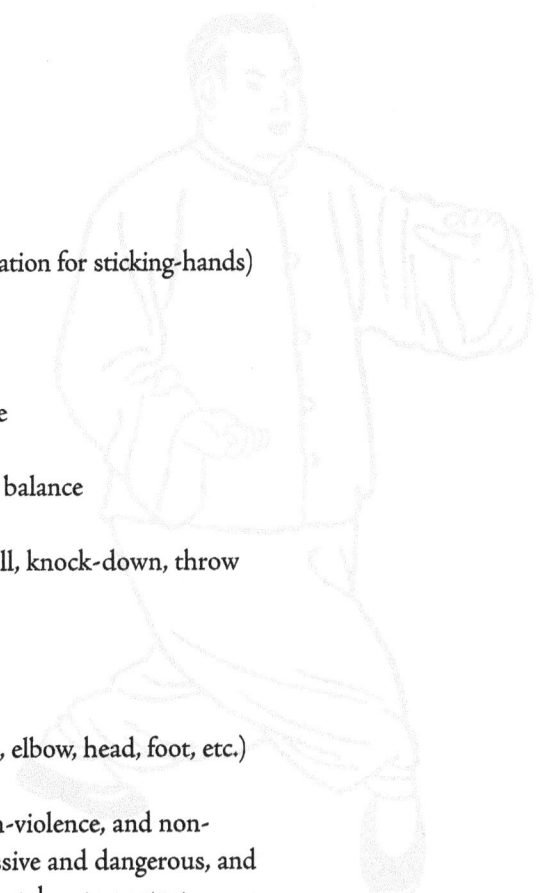

Health

For health, the Solo Form gives us relaxation, balance, flexibility, strength, and breath control. The pushing-hands will take all these actions further by gently challenging these areas. For example, you gain a certain degree of strength and flexibility in your legs and waist when you shift back in a stance. When someone is pushing you, you end up continually going a little past your limit, which will gradually increase that limit. During pushing-hands, your partner will push and pull you into places and positions that the Solo Form does not. The added bending, turning and moving can only be done softly, which will increase your degree of relaxation.

Another point is that having someone in your face, in your living space, pushing you, can be a real challenge to your breathing, mental calm, and centeredness. When you go back to Solo Form practice, you will notice how much deeper your relaxation, flexibility, etc. has become.

Self-Defense

For self-defense, pushing-hands gives us the basics for fighting skills, but is not the final answer. The most important skill is a developed sense of touch. The old adage, "the hand is quicker than the eye," means for us that an opponent may easily fool our eyes as to what they intend to do, but will find difficulty hiding the feelings of their intended attack.

The old masters called the sense of touch "listening energy (ting-jin)," like they could hear your actions and movements with their skin. The T'ai-Chi Classics tell us that after you can listen to energy, gradually you will be able to interpret the energy (tung-jin) as to how it will manifest itself, such as long or short, fast or slow, internal or external.

Master Liang always stressed that "to know before the action" was the way to mount a suitable defense. He broke an attack into three easy-to-understand time frames: before you are attacked, as you are attacked, and after you are attacked. Two of these you can defend against, but one is definitely too late.

There are five training words or phrases that help us develop our sense of touch and are commonly called the *five elements of pushing-hands*. All teachers have their own ways of describing them, so I will give you my brief ideas on each one.

Adhere is like when you glue two pieces of wood together. You have to use a clamp to make the glue effective. This word means to me: active sticking. I have to use some of my energy to stick to my partners so I can listen to

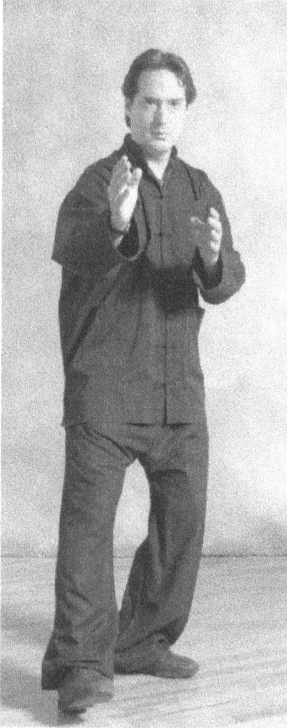

Paul Abdella demonstrates Lift Hands.

him. In other words, I am responsible for the work of sticking to my partner. Grandmaster Wai-lun Choi calls this "chasing" the hands.

Join is the action, or struggle, to keep connected to your partner so you can sense him. Either at the first moment or if he's trying to disconnect, join is the energy of getting back into contact. "Charging forward to stick and defend" is a funny way Master Liang used to describe join.

Stick is passive or staying easily in contact, feeling the opponent's power as it comes to you and avoiding it.

Follow is to be second or to take cues from your partner as to whether to go forward or backward, fast or slow, high or low. The *Tao Te Ching* says, "It is better to retreat one foot than to advance one inch, better to be the host than the guest." When someone is attacking, he has to take into account all your possible reactions, while the defender just has the attack to deal with. Follow means obey, listen to your opponent and obey him when he is telling you what his weak points are and how to defeat them.

No resistance, no letting go is what Master Liang called the "mother of the five elements" and the foundation for developing the sense of touch. Resistance can mean pushing at the exact same time as your partner. Letting go is breaking apart or having your partner escape your radar-like detection. Simply put, you can't feel anything, or feel correctly, in either situation.

Philosophy

The philosophy of T'ai-Chi, also called mental accomplishment or development, is based on the yin-yang symbol, which sums up the powers of active, passive, and neutral. An excellent definition of T'ai-Chi or yin and yang is opposites that cannot exist apart. The pushing-hands exercises thoroughly explore all manner of opposites, such as attack and defense, forward and backward, lead and follow, tension and relaxation, give and take, etc.

The *Tao Te Ching*, the handbook of Taoism and the wellspring of T'ai-Chi, advocates yielding, softness, and water to balance or overcome aggression, hardness, and stone. We can experience these thoughts or ideas physically as well as intellectually and emotionally with a partner.

We can actively experiment with softness to balance hardness, etc. It is easy to read a book or sit on a cushion or live in a cave and say, "I'm so spiritual, compassionate, caring, gentle and yielding," and then someone bumps into you or cuts you off on the highway and you explode into a raging, homicidal maniac. Pushing-hands practice with a live, thinking, breathing partner gives you plenty of hands-on practice and experience for putting Taoist philosophy into action.

Meditation

T'ai-Chi for meditation uses 70% Taoist and 30% Buddhist methods.

The Taoist method is about saving and storing energy, circulating and extending the energy, and balancing and controlling energy. In the Solo Form, we try to extend the energy out to the surface of the skin. This will give us complete circulation of blood, ch'i, and spirit. The practice of swimming in air helps to achieve this. In weapons training, we use the body, mind and eye to extend our energy and sense of touch by using the tip of the weapon as a concentration point. This practices extending through an inanimate object. In pushing-hands, we can extend our energy from our body out to five feet away by using a biological conduit — our partner's body. We can extend through their arms, torso, and legs down to the floor.

The Buddhist method is about emptiness, egolessness, and stopping the repetition of destructive habits. Many times during pushing-hands practice Master Liang would say, "Invest in loss," "Yield," "Don't take the initiative," and "Small loss, small gain; big loss, big gain." Pushing-hands practice done correctly can help us empty ourselves of ego, pride, and selfishness. We must learn to work with different people, adapt and change, and get along so our selves, our partners, our class, our families, and our world can survive in balance and harmony.

Enough preaching.

WHEN TO LEARN PUSHING-HANDS

As to when to start learning pushing-hands, I'll give a few examples. When Master Liang was learning from Cheng Man-ch'ing, Liang was recovering from liver disease. Cheng made Liang wait close to six years before he would let him do pushing-hands because he was concerned about any possible injury to a weakened internal organ. As for me, because I had asthma and allergies growing up, Master Liang made me wait two years, until he was sure my lungs were healthy.

I don't want to paint the picture of pushing-hands being so rough or violent. When you do pushing-hands, the whole body is affected and actually benefits from the contact. Because the torso is moved by someone else's energy, the safety precaution is only for people with a history of a weak or injured internal organ.

My generation of students was taught single-hand and four-directions pushing hands at the end of the second section of the Solo Form. (This was only practiced slow and soft, in the same vein as the Solo Form.) At our studio, the only prerequisite is the 150-posture Solo Form before you start pushing-hands classes. This way you'll have health and correct body knowledge, and will know many of the techniques used.

My personal opinion is that once you begin, you should continue with some aspect of pushing-hands for the rest of your life, but at the very least, one year of continuous training will benefit your T'ai-Chi.

How to Learn Pushing-Hands

Just as a great dish needs a recipe or an extensive trip needs a map, so too does the path of learning and practicing need a plan of action. T'ai-Chi as a system has many clear-cut formulae that we can use for learning and practicing as well as teaching. We are going to look at the T'ai-Chi symbol, which is a guideline for breaking down any learning/practicing plan into three parts. We will also use the eight trigrams, which will give us a couple of lesson plans in increments of eight.

When looking at the T'ai-Chi symbol, most people see black and white fish or dots, and this makes them think of opposites. But the symbol represents not just opposites, and not two, but three, powers: active, passive, and neutral. The three powers, called San-Tsai in Chinese, represent heavenly power, earthly power, and human power. If we approach pushing-hands in three progressive steps, we can not only save time and energy, but also understand pushing-hands and the system of T'ai-Chi as a whole.

The first set of three for learning is to train the body to become first soft, then hard, and then have the ability to freely change between the two. The T'ai-Chi Classics say, "From the most soft and yielding you will arrive at the most powerful and unyielding," and an old martial arts saying tells us to be able to make our bodies soft as cotton or as hard as steel in the blink of an eye. I can't emphasize enough that softness is not only one-third of the mastery of pushing-hands, but it must be the first part mastered.

Another set of three for learning purposes is the concept of *hua* (defend), *na* (control), and *da* (attack). Each technique in T'ai-Chi has three distinct parts which, at the highest level, are done together, but for learning purposes are mainly broken down into three parts. Defense can be defined as the many ways to avoid or reduce your partner's energy or attack from coming toward your body. Control is to stop any further energy coming from your partner. Attack is to issue your energy to your partner.

The first step in learning any pushing-hands practice is to study the defensive part, to truly understand how to protect yourself. Control is a very subtle idea of doing something to stop your partner from doing anything further to you after you have neutralized the first push or attack. This can be achieved by unbalancing, trapping, locking a joint or any number of other ways to try to freeze them, so to speak. Attack is to issue energy of your own for a specific counter-attack such as a push, strike, throw, trip, or a finishing joint lock.

When you understand the three parts of a technique separately, you can begin to combine them together. First, you should combine the defensive and controlling aspects and then counterattack, combining the three parts into two. The final stage is to defend, control, and counter in the same movement. Easy to say (or write), but difficult to do without years of correct practice.

There are many ways to use the three powers for training, but I'll just give one more. When learning a new method or practicing a familiar one, put your attention first on your body, then on your partner's body, and lastly on both bodies at the same time. Master Liang always told us, "The first step of pushing-hands is to make a thorough investigation of feeling and sensitivity." When practicing pushing-hands, I want to feel my body — Is it relaxed? Unified? Balanced? Am I in a defect position? Then, I want to feel my partner's body for the same qualities. Finally, I want to feel both our bodies at the same time, processing information and acting accordingly.

A common pitfall is to focus on your partner's faults and mistakes without first correcting your own. Without fail, 90% of all complaints made to me about other students are after a pushing-hands class. You work on getting yourself right. When that is done, you can look at and study your partner. Then, and only then, can you begin to understand any given technique from both points of view. *The Art of War* says, "To know yourself and know your opponent is to have 100 victories in 100 battles."

Eight Energies

There are many talks by different masters and authors about the 8 Postures of T'ai-Chi. These 8 Postures or Energies play an important role in pushing-hands. In Master Liang's book, *T'ai-Chi Ch'uan for Health and Self-Defense*, on pg. 89 the Classic says, "In Ward Off, Roll Back, Press, and Push one must know the correct technique." In the commentary it says, "They are supplemented by the movements of the four corners — Pull, Split, Elbow and Shoulder. Together, all of these are called the 8 positions (essences) and all the variations in T'ai-Chi Ch'uan are derived from them." The 8 Postures are not static or just single movements, they are actually outward manifestations of 8 intrinsic energies.

Here is a brief list with basic descriptions of the 8 Postures and the uses of the energy.

Ward Off: Keep out or away using the circular principle of the horizontal wheel (this is commonly the first energy to master).

Roll Back: Lead in and past, or away, like a matador with a bull (for Cheng Man-ch'ing, this was the first energy to master).

Press: One hand controls as the other hand counters.

Push: Manipulating yin and yang to attack partner's balance, control and attack with the same hand.

Pull: To guide the power or to off-balance, as if plucking fruit.

Split: Divide four options: split the power, break the joint, attack the stance, and split the mind from the body.

Elbow: All strikes, folding, and unfolding.

Shoulder: Short power.

The 8 Postures are, in essence, 8 sensations or feelings you develop within your body, manifested from your body to your partner's body, or sensed in your partner's body. The 8 Energies are one of the steps in understanding Master Liang's quote, "The first step of pushing-hands is to make a thorough investigation of feeling and sensibility."

Eight Conditions

When practicing pushing-hands with Master Liang, he would always remark that we didn't know him, but he knew us quite well. I found out later he was paraphrasing a line from the Classics that goes, "My opponent does not know me, but I know them quite well. If you can master all the techniques, you will become a peerless hero."

I asked him, "What is it that you know, that I don't know?" He answered, "The 8 Techniques." The word "techniques" confused me for many years because I thought of the word as related to physical procedures like blocks, grabs, attacks, etc.

Once I had grasped the 8 Techniques, I started calling them the 8 Conditions in my mind, and that cleared them up for my own learning, practice, and now, I hope, teaching. The 8 Techniques are essentially conditions present in your and your partner's bodies that make your attack effective, or his ineffective.

Here is a brief list of the 8 Techniques with basic descriptions:

Yin and Yang: The hard and soft, the insubstantial and substantial, the moving and the still and all the variations in between.

The Line: This is the weak point in your partner's stance or position and the direction that is the most effective for attacking it.

The Center of Gravity/Center Line: These are the horizontal and vertical lines in a person's torso that make it difficult for him to turn or defend himself.

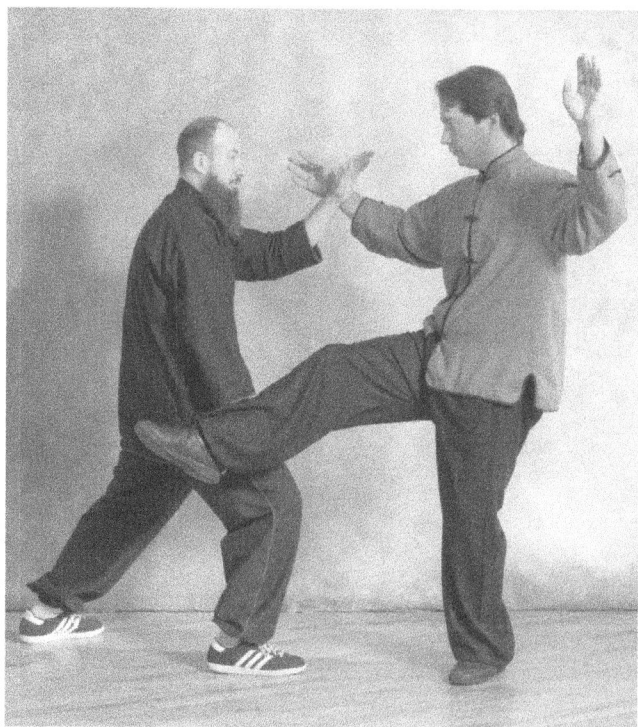

Ray Hayward and Paul Abdella practicing San-Shou.

Superior and Defect Position: Having your opponent at a disadvantage and being able to take advantage of it.

Single Weighting: Knowing the correct way to issue energy from your body.

Concentration of Energy: Like a mathematical equation, getting the whole body to issue energy at the same time for maximum power.

Control: The Chinese word na, which means to seize or hold, the technique of keeping your opponent in the defect position.

Territory: The "living space" of your and your partner's stance — how to get inside your partner's territory to attack without him taking advantage of you.

Master Liang told me that the Yang family could get all 8 Conditions any time they wanted and that is why their pushing-hands was so effective. He also said to work on one or two and gradually build up to getting all eight before pushing. There are numerous references made about the 8 Techniques/Conditions in Master Liang's book — see pp. 5, 24, 26, 39, 41, 76 and 91.

EIGHT LEVELS

In my early days studying with Master Liang, I loved to ask him questions and hear his stories and comments about the old masters, especially the Yang family. One day I asked a question that elicited an answer which, to this day, continually gives me fresh insight. I asked Master Liang, "At what level are you, compared to Cheng Man-ch'ing and the Yang family?" He answered by saying, "I asked Professor Cheng the very same question."

Master Liang was told what the various levels were and how to recognize them. He alluded to these levels on page 105 in the short text called "To Know Before the Action" in his book, which states, "The way of T'ai-Chi can be divided into three levels: that of one who has foresight and vision, one who knows and apprehends only after the event, and one who knows nothing from beginning to end. As soon as fellow disciples of T'ai-Chi join hands and begin to practice the pushing-hands exercise, they can perceive each other's level of mastery."

I like to tell students that when you meet a new partner for pushing-hands, you want to figure out — Is this person more, less, or the same level of sensitivity? If more, work on defense. If less, work on offense. If equal, work on sensitivity, which is all the variations of yin and yang.

As T'ai-Chi for health, self-defense, philosophy, and meditation are all based on the nervous system, or more simply, the sense of touch, we can see the correlation between how delicate and refined the sense of touch is and how elevated the level of martial ability and meditation.

Once again, here are the 8 Levels, brief descriptions, and a reference to each from the Classics:

Jumping Energy (*t'iao-chin*): When your partner's energy has fully reached your body, you "ride" it and land safely, maintaining your relaxation and centeredness. "When you have been struck and are just about to fall over, you must hop like a sparrow."

Neutralizing Energy (*hua-chin*): When your partner's energy is 70% in your body, you turn, shift, bend, etc. to neutralize, reduce or transform it so that you maintain your balance. "When your partner puts pressure on the left, the left becomes insubstantial; when pressure is brought on the right, the right becomes empty."

Withdraw/Attack Energy (*tsou fa chin*): When your opponent's energy comes to your body, you neutralize it, borrow some of it, and issue energy of your own at the same instant. "To withdraw is to attack; to attack is to withdraw."

Receiving Energy (*chieh-chin*): When your opponent has issued half his energy, you combine the skills of neutralizing, rooting, and issuing with timing and sensitivity to add your push to the last half of his push — getting 150% by spending 100%. "Suddenly disappear and suddenly appear."

Listening Energy (*t'ing-chin*): The sense of touch is so developed at this stage that as soon as your partner's muscles are stirring with energy, about to push you, you can feel it or "hear it coming" and push first, anticipating and stopping him. "If your opponent does not move, you do not move. At the slightest stir, you have already anticipated it and moved beforehand."

Interpreting Energy (*tung-chin*): Akin to Chinese medicine, you can feel which organ/meridian is manifesting energy and know, or interpret, which action the person is taking, be it offensive, defensive, or controlling, before the muscles even move. "From the mastery of all the postures, you will apprehend 'interpreting energy;' from apprehending interpreting energy, you will arrive at a complete mastery of your partner without recourse to detecting his energy."

Sticking Energy (*nien-chin*): By controlling positive and negative charges in the body, the practitioner can attract or repel a partner using bioelectric magnetic energy. "The mind and the ch'i must respond ingeniously and efficaciously to the exchange of substantial and insubstantial so as to develop an active and harmonious tendency."

Spiritual Insight (*shen-ming*): The practitioner's sense of touch is so acute that he can feel/read the intentions of a partner and anticipate them well in advance — "reading his mind" and dealing with the attack perfectly. "After you have learned to interpret energy, the more you practice, the better your skill will be, and by examining thoroughly and remembering silently, you will gradually reach a stage of total reliance on the mind."

As we can see from this list, the 8 Levels are about how sensitive your nervous system is and at what distance your nervous system becomes aware. Master Liang said, "When you practice the Solo Form, imagine you are swimming in air. This will make your body so sensitive and alert. Gradually, you will become aware of an ever-increasing area around your body."

These three lists of eight are considered by many masters to be the "secrets" of T'ai-Chi Ch'uan, and they would make their students wait many years before revealing them, if ever.

As we can see, the secret is not in what we do, but in how we do it. A Classic says, "To enter the gate and be guided onto the correct path, one requires verbal instruction from a competent master. If one practices constantly and studies carefully, one's skill will take care of itself." Master Liang, in his true role as a teacher, learned them, cataloged them, taught them, explained them, demonstrated the ones he could, and encouraged us to seek the highest levels.

I've said it before and I'll say it again: the first, last and always starting point to any pushing-hands practice is softness, but I'll let the Classics sum up this whole article: "From the most soft and yielding you will arrive at the most powerful and unyielding."

Pushing-Hands: Just One Aspect of Self-Defense

Ray Hayward

This article appeared in **T'ai-Chi — Perspectives of the Way and its Movement,** *Vol. 9, No. 1, February 1985, published by Wayfarer Publications, Los Angeles.*

Is there too much emphasis on pushing-hands? The answer to this question is yes. Pushing-hands is only the second step of a four-step process we go through to acquire the art of T'ai-Chi Ch'uan for self-defense. The first step is equilibrium. The second is pushing-hands. The third is free-hand. The fourth is weapons training.

Now let me briefly explain each step so we can see what each has to contribute to our self-defense training. The first step, equilibrium, is also called "getting a root." When we practice T'ai-Chi Ch'uan, we must pay extra attention to our steps. When we step with one foot, it should be empty; then we should gradually shift our weight to that foot.

Achieving a Root is Essential

In this way, we can fully exercise our legs and gain enough flexible strength to be able to "root." If you step with weight on both feet, you will be committing the mistake of "double-weighting" and will be taken far off the path to equilibrium.

When you have gained a root, no one can push you over, no matter what technique they use. You have the energy to resist, but won't, and can neutralize an opponent's energy because your waist can obey your mind.

If you don't have a root, when you turn your waist to neutralize, you will fall over by your action. Without a root, you won't be able to apply the subtle techniques of T'ai-Chi Ch'uan. So this can be considered the most important step.

The second step, pushing-hands, can be divided into two parts. The first part is learning how to yield. This is for defense. We want to lose, not gain — small loss, small gain; big loss, big gain. When we are pushed, we don't resist.

Pushed 100 Times, Yield 100 Times

If we can't neutralize, we just fall over without a struggle. This is called "investing in loss," which rids us of our ego and fully exercises our legs to further develop our root.

Gradually, we will be able to neutralize and not let our opponent's energy come to our bodies. If we are pushed 100 times, we will yield 100 times, never losing balance. We are like willow trees, bending 100 times in the wind. Our waist seems "boneless." Once you reach this stage, you can go on to learn the second part of pushing-hands: counter-attack.

To counter-attack the opponent is not so easy. You must know the techniques of insubstantial and substantial, and the techniques of finding the center of gravity, and finding your opponent's defect position while maintaining your superior position. You must also know the most effective line to push the opponent, and how to concentrate your energy in one direction while avoiding "double-weighting."

You must not collide with your opponent. You must know about all the kinds of energies, such as withdraw-attack energy, uprooting energy, "on the spot" energy, sudden energy, neutralizing energy, hearing energy, receiving energy, interpreting energy, and the sticking energy as used by the Yang family.

There are many more kinds of energy, but all of them come from using the whole body as one unit. If you don't have all of these conditions before you counter-attack the opponent, you will fall into the error of "double-weighting" and only execute a "blind push." Only these techniques can be considered the true way of counter-attacking in T'ai-Chi Ch'uan.

The Third Step

The third step, free-hand, can also be divided into two parts: Ta-Lu and sparring sets. Ta-Lu is an advanced practice in which two people use the original 13 postures to attack and defend.

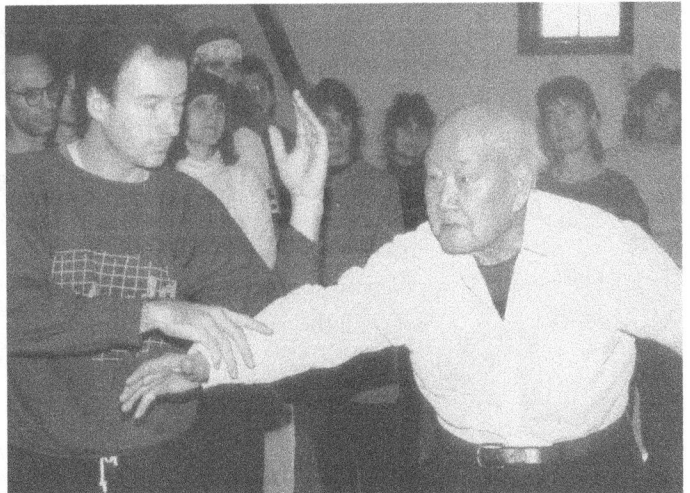

Ray Hayward and Master T.T. Liang demonstrate San-Shou at Paul Gallagher's Deer Mountain Taoist Academy Workshop and Seminar in 1988.

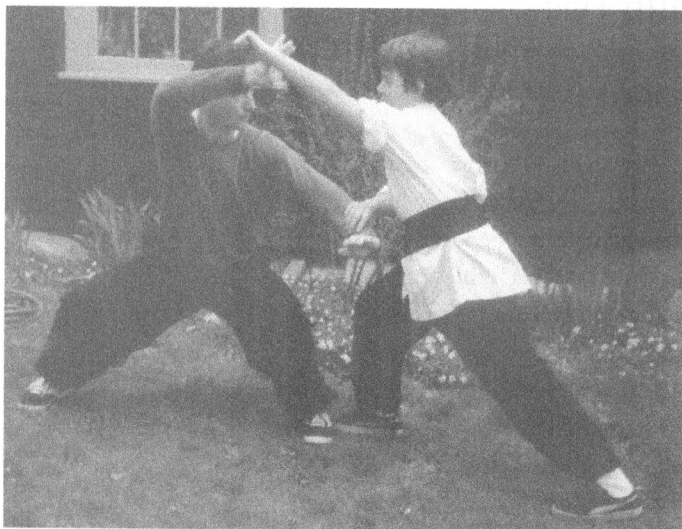

Ray Hayward and J. Richard Roy's son, Travis, practicing Pa Kua at J.R. Roy's home in Greenfield, Massachusetts in 1983.

Ta-Lu helps the practitioner to further understand the neutralizing, pushing, and striking techniques as well as how to utilize the five steps and the eight directions. An example is the Yang family's Ta-Lu, which uses the techniques of Roll Back, Push, Shoulder, and Slap, following the eight directions.

Wang Yen-nien's Ta-Lu uses Ward Off, Roll Back, Push, and Press against Pull, Split, Elbow, and Shoulder following an East-West direction.

The sparring sets, also called "miscellaneous combat," use the postures from the Solo Form as well as auxiliary techniques to show how the principles of T'ai-Chi Ch'uan are used to handle counter-punching and kicking attacks as well as pushing and grappling attacks.

Included in every posture are the three techniques of *hua*/neutralize, *na*/hold, and *da*/attack. The sets also teach how to "join" with an opponent, and how to 'stick' with them so you can sense their intentions. You also review all the pushing-hands techniques as well as learn how to "change steps" and "turn body." You learn various "folding" techniques as well as how to control your opponent.

Without learning the third step, it will be difficult to engage in combat with opponents from other martial arts systems. It should be noted that my teacher, T.T. Liang, combined all the pushing-hands, Ta-Lus, and sparring sets into one form he calls the T'ai-Chi two-person dance. By practicing one round of this form, which has 178 postures, students can cover all the aspects of the two-person training.

THE FOURTH STEP

The fourth step, weapons training, is very important to the development of the intrinsic energy. By practicing the empty-hand forms, we are starting to develop the intrinsic energy, but by practicing with weapons, we can fully develop our energy. Most martial arts strike out with the arm, which uses force from the bone. This force is exhaustible as well as detrimental to health. T'ai-Chi Ch'uan uses the intrinsic energy that comes from the sinews and tendons of the whole body. The added weight of the weapons helps to fully strengthen the sinews, which in turn strengthens the intrinsic energy.

When practicing empty-handed, we try to get our energy to our hands, but when using the weapons, we try to extend our energy to the very tip of the weapon. After practicing with weapons, we find it easier to get energy into our hands, and we find an increased amount of energy at our command.

So, the purpose of weapons training is to fully develop and liberate our intrinsic energy. If you don't have this energy, you won't be able to apply the techniques of T'ai-Chi Ch'uan and will never advance even to the lowest levels.

In conclusion, let me say that the reason some modern practitioners can't use their art for self-defense is because they haven't followed the correct procedure of learning and practicing. Equal attention must be given to the four steps. Not one may be missing.

Ray Hayward demonstrates Raise the Bamboo Curtain from T'ai-Chi Sword.

Let us remember the Yang family and their disciples, who depended solely on T'ai-Chi Ch'uan for their self-defense skills. All the aforementioned information was told and taught to me by my master, Liang Tung-tsai. My deepest thanks go to him.

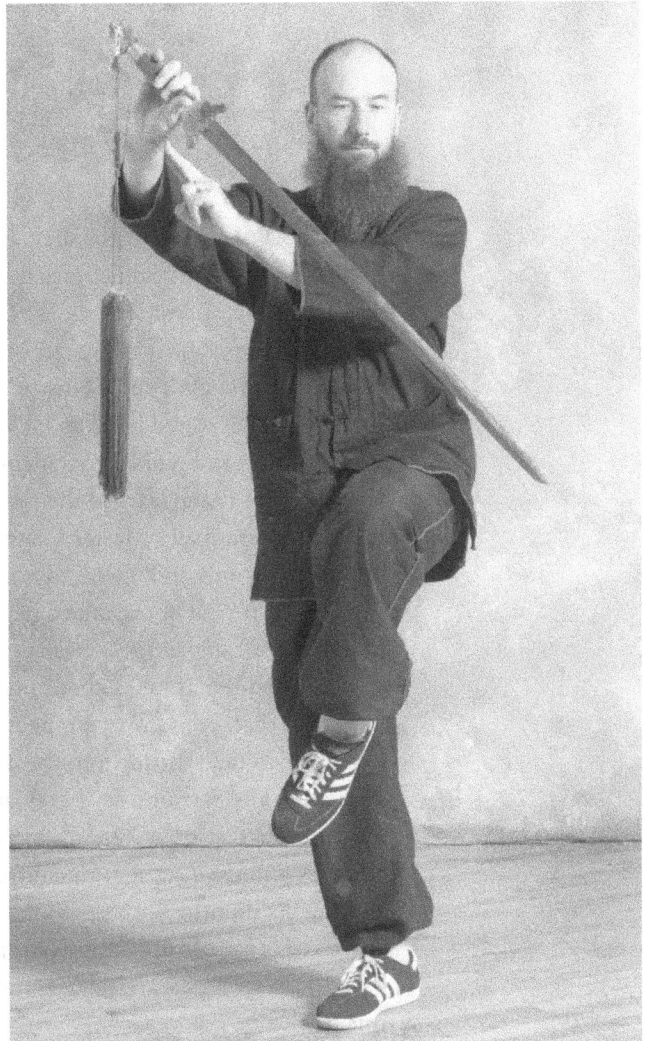

SAN-SHOU:
A SHORT HISTORY

RAY HAYWARD

In the T'ai-Chi Ch'uan system, there is a two-person form called San-Shou or "free-hand." Sometimes it is called "miscellaneous combat." Master T.T. Liang referred to it as the T'ai-Chi 2-Person Dance, or just as "the dance." To him, dancing is an act of cooperation, and he felt that the two-person form taught people how to cooperate with each other.

San-Shou, created by Yang Chien-hou, is an advanced progression from pushing and pulling to punching, kicking, knockdowns and joint locks. Master Liang learned the San-Shou from Master Hsiung Yang-hou in Taiwan. Gradually, Master Liang added the other two-person practices of pushing-hands and Ta-Lu to make his 178-posture two-person dance.

On a historical note, some of the postures in the San-Shou are not found in the Yang-style Solo Form, but are from the original Chen style.

At the studio, it takes about one year to learn the 178 movements. We have seen that, year after year, people complete one side, but really don't have time to take the form to the deeper levels. Paul and I have been discussing and working to abbreviate the San-Shou back to its original length, which is about 72 movements. We are going to experiment for one year and try a six-month course to learn the shortened version, and another six months for corrections, principles and advanced studies. We will try this for the upcoming year and if it doesn't work well, we will go back to the 178-posture sequence and try another method for teaching this level.

Weapons Training:
History, Theory, and Benefits

Ray Hayward

In recent years, we have taught many people solo and two-person weapons. We have received requests for some in-depth knowledge and history about weapons and their usage. There are many reasons for weapons training and many solo and two-person weapon methods. I will try to cover three areas in this article. The first part will be a basic history and evolution of the weapons, the second some theories and principles, and the third will examine the benefits of weapons training.

History

The history of weapons is as old as humanity. Weapons were originally needed for survival and later for warfare; their modern uses, as in our case, they are for health training and sport.

The earliest weapons were clubs, which evolved with the addition of various spikes. Then the spikes evolved to short blades, which became axes. As ax blades became longer and handles became shorter, the sabre or broadsword evolved. These kinds of weapons were primarily swung and relied upon the weight of the weapon and the strength of the arm of the wielder.

The second source of weapons was the stick or staff. Made of various lengths and held in two hands, it evolved to have a simple sharpened point, then to stone or steel heads affixed to one end. Thus the spear was born. Spears were made in many different ways. Some had ax-like blades or hooks attached to the sides, others were made of various lengths, and still others had varied shapes of points or spearheads.

Gradually the spearhead became longer

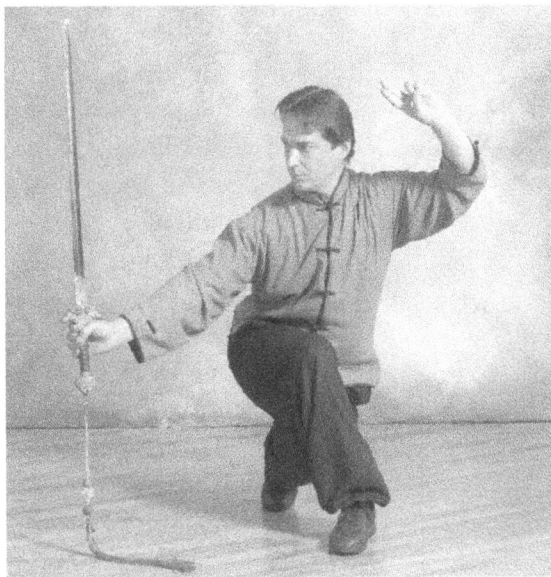

Paul Abdella demonstrates the Planting Lotus Flowers Upside-Down posture from the Tamo Sword form with tassel.

and the handle became shorter so the spear could be wielded with one hand. This weapon gradually evolved to be the double-edged sword. This kind of weapon was primarily pushed or thrust toward the opponent, using parrying and dodging for defense and relying on speed and agility as opposed to brute strength.

There is a saying in T'ai-Chi: "If you swing the double-edged sword like the sabre, then the founder of T'ai-Chi will laugh at you from his grave." This shows that one must understand the differences in use, method, and power source between these two weapons.

In Chinese martial arts, there are many references to the four major weapons: the staff, the sabre, the spear and the sword. The staff and the sabre are called the "hard" weapons; the sword and the spear are called the "soft" weapons. The hard weapons are those that are heavy in weight, use blocks for defense, and generally require a reasonable degree of strength. The soft weapons are lighter and flexible. They use more parrying, sticking and dodging for defense, and they rely on speed and footwork to be effective.

There are many other weapons such as flexible weapons, double weapons, and various long and short weapons. In T'ai-Chi, we use three weapons: the sword, the sabre and the spear.

THEORY

In this section, I'd like to explain three areas: the extension of ch'i, *hua-na-da*, and three kinds of energy.

In the T'ai-Chi Classics, there are many references to mind, ch'i, and the direction and extension of the ch'i or bio-energy:

"Let the mind direct the ch'i so that it sinks deeply and steadily and can permeate the bones."

"To direct the ch'i is like threading a pearl with nine crooked paths."

"The mind is the leader and the body is the follower."

Master Liang has said, "If every movement can be directed by the mind-intent within and manifested without, then the internal spiritual aspect and external physical aspect will be united. Thus the body will instantly follow the dictates of the mind and the ch'i, and intrinsic energy will immediately reach the intended point."

Master Liang also told us, "When practicing T'ai-Chi sword, keep your eyes focused on the tip. This keeps the spirit of vitality alive and helps the mind-intent send the ch'i to the tip." "The reason we practice with weapons is so we can reach the tip with our ch'i. When we can direct energy to the tip of a weapon, it becomes easy to get it to circulate to the hands." "You have to learn to extend your energy, to go from the body to the hand and out to the tip of the weapon."

And lastly from Master Liang, "Weapons training becomes more important than empty hand training only after you can circulate energy to the hands."

From the Classics and from the teachings of Master Liang, we can see that weapons training is really for the circulation, direction, and extension of our mind and energy.

In T'ai-Chi Ch'uan as a martial art, each single technique can be broken down into three components. The first part of any technique is *hua*. *Hua* means to neutralize or transform. This is the defensive aspect. The second component, *na*, means to seize or hold. This is for controlling the opponent by offsetting his balance or trapping his limbs and body. The third aspect, *da*, literally means strike, but can also mean to issue your intrinsic energy. This is the counter-attacking part of the technique.

Master Liang has always said, "When the *hua-na-da* are separate, you are dancing with your partner. But when the three parts are done all at once, you will knock out your partner."

To train these three aspects, the Yang style uses three weapons: the sword, the saber and the spear. The sword corresponds to *hua*. The sword, using evasive and subtle defenses, utilizes *hua* to be effective. Thus we say that by training the sword we are strengthening the *hua* aspect of our training.

The saber utilizes *na*, or holding, to be effective. The drag step and the lunging and grabbing are ways that the saber trains the holding or controlling techniques. So we say that by training the saber we strengthen the *na* aspect of our training.

The spear corresponds to *da*. The spear uses direct strikes while using the follow step to illustrate the point that the best defense is offense. The length and weight of the spear require you to use your whole body when you issue energy. So we say that the spear strengthens the *da*.

From this example, we can see that the solo weapons each contribute to the self-defense aspects of the T'ai-Chi techniques. The old masters insisted that three kinds of energy must be developed. They felt that the energy must be directed first in a straight line, then on a plane, and finally, at the highest level, on a pinpoint. This means that the mind would direct the energy, which would be projected out of the body in one of these three ways.

The first way of issuing energy, which is a straight line, is to learn how to use the body as one unit and project the energy straight out from your body. When we train with the spear, this is the kind of energy we use. The spear helps to develop straight-line energy.

The second way we learn to issue energy is across a horizontal plane. This requires training in the waist and legs. The saber uses this kind of energy; thus, the saber will help to train your energy to project out on a horizontal plane.

The highest level is pinpoint energy, where all the body's energy is focused to a very small area. Because we focus on the tip of the sword, this kind of energy is naturally developed through sword practice. The sword uses many pinpoint techniques such as *dien*, which means pointing, and *peng*, which means snapping. These techniques clearly show the body energy focused through the weapon to a very small area. So we say that the sword helps to train pinpoint energy.

Benefits

In this section, I will explain some of the benefits and lessons of weapons training.

To practice T'ai-Chi without weapons is to strengthen the muscles of the body, and to practice T'ai-Chi with weapons is to strengthen the sinews and bones. When practicing T'ai-Chi with weapons, the body, the hands and the weapon should act as one unit so that the intrinsic energy will reach to the tip of the weapon.

~ *Liang Tung-tsai*

From the above quote from our teacher, we can see that the weapons play an important part in the strengthening process of T'ai-Chi. The weapons are our "weight-lifting," so to speak, but we want strong sinews, ligaments, tendons, and bones as well as strong and supple muscles. The Solo Form and pushing-hands are enough to strengthen the legs and waist, although the more advanced stances and footwork of the weapons forms can still further exercise our lower bodies. The weapons mainly give

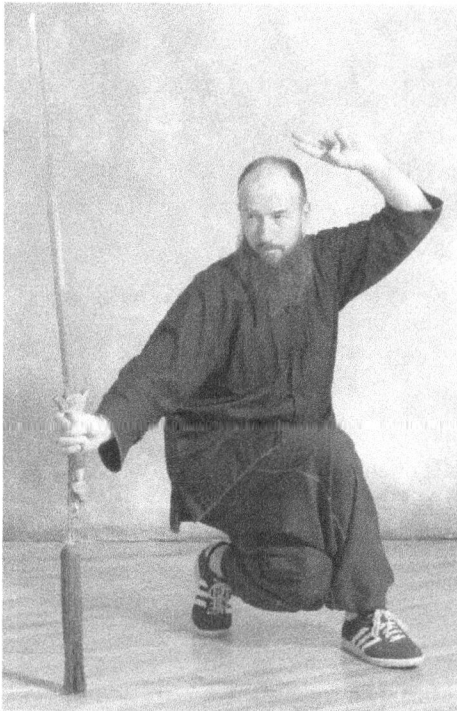

Ray Hayward demonstrates the Planting Lotus Flowers Upside-Down posture from the Tamo Sword form with tassel.

us our upper-body workout.

All the weapons have the benefit of strengthening the fingers and hands. The sword, with its intricate angles and circles, works the wrist and upper arm. The knife, or sabre, by using large sweeping movements, exercises the upper arm and shoulder. The spear, with its added length and weight, strengthens the shoulders and back. Of course, the weapons are to be wielded by the entire body, which gets exercised, but these areas receive more attention and benefit.

It is said that the sword corresponds to the sword-hand strike, also called the Immortal Strike, which uses the index and middle finger joined together to strike at vulnerable points. The sword form strengthens this hand position. The knife corresponds to the knife hand, the James Bond karate chop, and helps develop that strike. The spear corresponds to the spear hand, or the thrusting hand, which uses all the fingers to stab the opponent. The spear movements help strengthen this strike. (On a side note, the staff corresponds to the fist and helps develop punching techniques.)

There is also the Theory of Refinement for the weapons. The sword is said to refine the spirit and feeling, the knife refines the footwork, and the spear refines the ability to issue energy (*fa-ching*). The weapons also factor in the theory of Taoist alchemy. The spear changes *ching*, or sexual energy, to ch'i, or breath energy. The knife changes ch'i to *shen*, or spirit. And the sword changes shen to *hsu*, or emptiness.

I see the weapons as the Taoists' revenge. Taoism is a pacifist religion/philosophy based on harmony and balance of opposites. The Taoists took instruments of killing and destruction and used them for the purposes of building health and strength, cultivating spirit, and expressing a moving art form. They could have easily exercised with brooms, shovels, bricks or ladles.

I'd like to end this article with an observation made years ago while watching a movie of Professor Cheng Man-ching demonstrating the Solo Form and the sword form. After the movie, we asked Master Liang why Professor Cheng's Solo Form and sword form, although both were relaxed, looked so different to us. They were both T'ai-Chi forms and the same person was performing them, so why would the energies look so different? Master Liang answered, saying, "Because in the Solo Form, Professor Cheng worked with the principles, but in the sword form, he played with the principles."

STRETCHING FOR LIFE: AN INTRODUCTION TO STRETCHING METHODS

Paul Abdella

The benefits of regular stretching are known to most people; however, many people do not know that virtually all methods of stretching can be placed in one of three general categories: relaxed stretching, dynamic stretching, and isometric stretching.

These stretching categories are distinguished by how they attempt to alter or reset the stretch reflex when a muscle is stretched. What is the stretch reflex? Here is an example that we've all probably experienced.

It's the end of a physically active day and you decide to do a little stretching before bed. You prepare yourself to do some toe touches; feet apart, straighten the legs, bend forward from the waist, lower yourself down and then — thud, your palms touch the floor. Wow! Amazing! You've never stretched that far before!

You hold the stretch a few seconds and feel a warm tingling tautness at the back of your legs that skirts the edge between pain and pleasure. You rise up slightly, then lower yourself down again. This time you feel a deeper release in the muscles as you drop to a little lower position. You hang timeless, like a cloud in space, until your body informs you that it's time to stop. You stand up, shake your legs out a little, and retire to bed, completely satisfied.

The next day you leap out of bed ready to repeat last night's performance in your morning routine. You loosen the neck and shoulders a little, rotate the trunk and hips, perform a few more routine warm-ups then ready yourself for toe touches. You assume a proper stance, bend forward, lower down, and — OUCH! There's a tug on your hamstrings that pulls like a dog's leash. It stops you, barely halfway to the floor.

Surprised but determined, you rise up to try again — this time a little more forcefully. Although you manage to get a bit lower on the second try, the contraction at the back of your legs is sharper. It leaves a tingling residue of pain that causes you to stop and abandon the stretch — the same stretch that just hours before felt so free and natural. What happened? The activation of the stretch reflex.

The stretch reflex is a safety mechanism built into a muscle. When a muscle is stretched, special groups of cells called stretch receptors (contained in the muscle fibers) inform the central nervous system about their state of tension. This information is received by the central nervous system, which sends a message back to the muscle telling it to contract. This contraction acts as a brake on the muscle, preventing it from stretching too far and being injured.

In the case of the evening stretch, the muscles were warm and elastic, with plenty of blood flowing through them from a full day of activity. After receiving this information from the muscles, the central nervous system applied only a mild contraction, allowing a greater stretch to occur. It then released the contraction as the muscles relaxed more deeply, allowing for an even greater stretch.

In the case of the morning stretch, the muscles had been inactive for a period of several hours during sleep. When the attempt was made to touch the toes, the stretch reflex contracted the muscles firmly. This prevented them from lengthening too much before they were sufficiently warmed up.

As I stated earlier, the three general categories of stretching methods can be distinguished by how each attempts to reset or alter the stretch reflex to a lower tension level. This allows for a greater range of motion, with a reduced risk of injury. Let's take a look at each of these stretching categories in more detail.

Relaxed Stretching

Relaxed stretching is the most common and widely practiced form of stretching. It is characterized by slowly relaxing your body into a stretch and holding it there for a time. Imagine a ballerina with her leg held up to the barre,

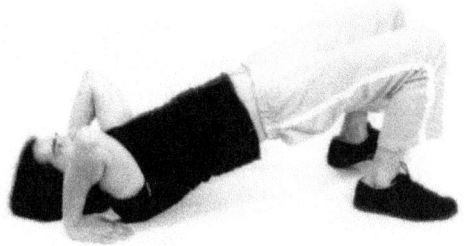

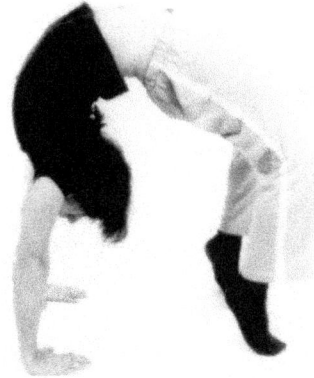

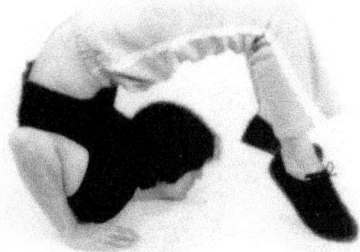

An extremely flexible Paul Abdella demonstrates a paricularly difficult stretch for an unpublished stretching book in 1980. Don't try this at home, kids!

gracefully lowering her rounded torso to it.

As the name implies, you assume positions that let you relax your muscles as you move into the stretch. You feel the tension in the muscles created by the stretch reflex. As you stretch, you move past the point of tension a little, hold, then move out of the stretch. As you repeat this sequence, eventually the stretch reflex is adjusted and the level of tension in the muscle lessens and you can ease into a new position.

Advantages: Relaxed stretching can be done anytime. It does not cause fatigue in the muscles, so you can do it when you are tired. It is the safest method of stretching, which makes it ideal to use when you are recovering from an injury. You will instinctively do relaxed stretching after being in one position for too long because it just plain feels good.

Limitations: Although it is the safest method of stretching to use, it is also the slowest to gain new levels of flexibility. Relaxed stretching also won't build strength in a muscle, as do other forms, and may even diminish it if done to an excessive degree.

Prescription: Do relaxed stretching before a workout, then afterward as a cool down. You can also use it as a counterbalance to fatigue, stress, or being in one position to long.

Dynamic Stretching

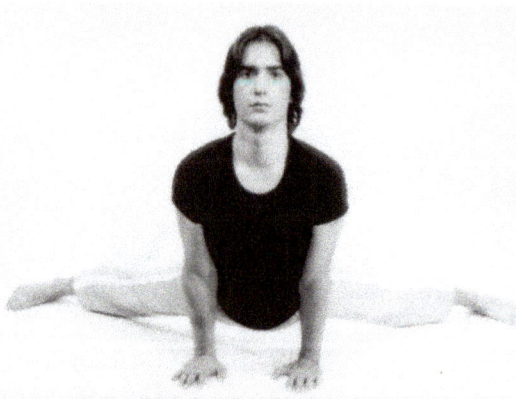

This stretch doesn't look too easy either! From the same unpublished book.

Dynamic stretching (sometimes called ballistic stretching) can be defined as a stretch or movement that is started by a muscular contraction but is completed by momentum. This momentum often takes the muscles outside a normal range of motion. Dynamic stretching most closely resembles the activities in which we all engage. Imagine a football kicker warming up to punt a ball with a few half-speed kicks in the air; a golfer gliding through a swing with an imaginary club; a baseball player loosening arm and shoulder with a relaxed throwing motion.

Contrary to current wisdom, dynamic

stretching is completely natural and safe if done properly. Begin by lightly swinging the limb to be stretched, and feel for the point of tension or resistance in the muscles. As the level of tension in the muscles decreases, you can increase the range of motion until you feel you've reached your maximum range. At this point, continue with a few more repetitions.

Stop before the muscles get fatigued. Muscles are less elastic when they are tired, so their ability to stretch is diminished. If you persist in doing dynamic stretches when your muscles are fatigued, you run the risk of resetting the stretch reflex back to a higher tension level.

Advantages: Dynamic stretching creates elasticity in the muscles, and if practiced consistently it can greatly reduce the time needed to warm-up before a workout.

Limitations: The effectiveness of dynamic stretching is reduced when muscles are tired. Also, if you stretch to your maximum range too quickly and forcefully using dynamic stretching, you may develop small tears or fissures in the muscle fiber, which will heal in a less elastic condition. This can inhibit your ability to gain the flexibility levels you desire.

Prescription: First, do a small amount of relaxed stretching to limber the joints, then do your dynamic stretches, followed by your workout. Include as many dynamic stretches that resemble movements in your sport or activity as you can.

Isometric Stretching

Isometric stretching is a form of stretching where a muscle is first stretched and then contracted against some form of resistance for a short period of time (about five seconds) before being released. This stretch, contract, release cycle is repeated from three to five times, increasing the stretch a little with each sequence until your maximum range of motion is achieved. The resistance is created by stretching and contracting against an immovable object and using a weight to apply force to the stretching muscles.

Again, imagine a dancer with her leg outstretched on the barre. This time she lowers the weight of her torso just to the first sign of tension in the stretched muscles. Then she contracts the stretched muscles at the back of her leg by pushing downward against the bar, holding this position

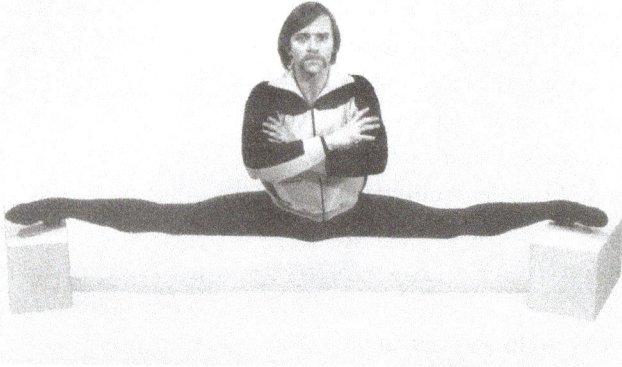

Doug Anderson (Paul's first stretching teacher) demonstrates a suspended side-split for an unpublished stretching book in 1980.

a few seconds and then releasing the contraction. She lowers her torso down a little further and repeats the sequence. With each stretch, contraction, and release, the muscle tension caused by the stretch reflex is lessened, creating a gain in flexibility.

Advantages: Isometric stretching is the fastest method of gaining new levels of flexibility in muscles. To contract a muscle with a load or weight on it is the basic principle in developing strength. This is why isometric stretching develops strength in a muscle throughout a full range of motion.

Limitations: To reap the greatest benefit and minimize any damage to your connective tissue, your muscles have to be healthy and strong to do isometric stretching.

Prescription: Isometric stretching works by activating the Golgi tendon reflex. This is a special stretch receptor located in the tendon and designed to pick up sensations of too much stretch or stress on the muscles. When activated, it overrides the muscle contractions caused by the stretch reflex and simply shuts the muscle down in order to protect the tendon from injury.

Because of this muscular shutdown, it's not good to do isometric stretching before or during your workout. Do isometric stretching right after your workout — two to four times per week in sets of three to five repetitions per muscle group. Hold each rep about five seconds. Hold the last rep a little longer — up to thirty seconds.

Regular stretching, along with aerobic and strength-building activities, will increase the muscles' normal resting length, making them more elastic and greatly reducing the risk of injury. Developing an awareness of tension levels in the muscles caused by the stretch reflex, plus an understanding of the three methods of stretching, will give you the ability to create a body equipped to perform at the levels you need, for a lifetime.

A Weekend with Master Wai-Lun Choi

Paul Abdella

In May 2002, Ray and I traveled to Chicago to visit Master Choi to continue our studies with him. I was interested in learning more of the Liu Ho Pa Fa Main Form and Ray was going to study more Pa-Kua and Hsing-I weapons.

We arrived at Master Choi's studio Saturday afternoon and found him watching a Chinese cable TV station, which was showing an interview with two distinguished academics. One was the head of a prestigious university in China, the other the head of Oxford University in England. A question was asked of the Chinese scholar: "What's the most important thing you teach the students at your university?" The professor answered, "Not to look and think in only a straight line, but rather to see and think with a broader field of vision." Master Choi exclaimed, "Good answer! Just like martial arts." He then spoke for the next 15 minutes on how this has been his objective in teaching "real internal training" for years. This discourse set the tone for an enjoyable and valuable weekend of study.

We began our session with Master Choi correcting my Main Form while Ray manned the video camera. Master Choi has considerable knowledge and skill in T'ai-Chi, Hsing-I, and Pa-Kua, but the Liu Ho Pa Fa Main Form is the crown jewel in his repertoire of styles. He knows every centimeter of the form in great detail and my form felt strong, natural, and comfortable after receiving the subtle corrections he made to it.

A review of the self-defense applications for the form came next. Many of the applications he demonstrated were different than those we had learned previously. When asked about this, Master Choi said since fighting is unpredictable, any given movement in a form should be applicable to different situations. The founder of the style had an idea in his mind that worked in his generation and we should analyze and adapt it, but "don't copy it." This means we must understand the principle in order to freely use it, as a situation demands.

Master Choi used the analogy of learning architecture by studying the blue print of a particular building. By only copying the blueprint, you continually build the same building over and over rather than understanding the principles of architecture and engineering to design original structures that fit their environment.

Ray and I changed roles as student and cameraman and a session of Pa-Kua and Hsing-I staff and spear techniques began. Every weapon is used in a particular way based on its physical design, but weapons must be thought of as an extension of the hand. Master Choi clearly demonstrated this idea through the 5 elements of Hsing-I and various Pa-Kua palm changes.

Our afternoon session came to a close all too quickly even though it was over three hours long. It was time for a well-deserved meal.

Master Choi drove us to our favorite Chinese restaurant in Chicago, Li Wing Wa in Chinatown. There he ordered in Cantonese the best beef and pan-fried noodles we've had anywhere, a delicious shrimp in honey-mustard sauce with glazed walnuts, and crispy chicken. The tea and conversation flowed as we waited for the food to be served. At one point Ray asked Master Choi what his Liu Ho Pa Fa teacher Chan Yik Yan's favorite food was. This brought up a story about a banquet that Master Choi held in his teacher's honor when he was a student.

Grandmaster Chan loved to eat fish, but his favorite fish was a large, rare and very expensive fish (he said the name in Chinese but not in English) that was considered a delicacy in Hong Kong. The fish needed to be caught and prepared the same day, and a special chef who knew how to cook it had to be used. To cover the cost, Choi and the guests had to pay a hundred dollars each — this was in the early 1960s. As a self-employed truck driver, the time

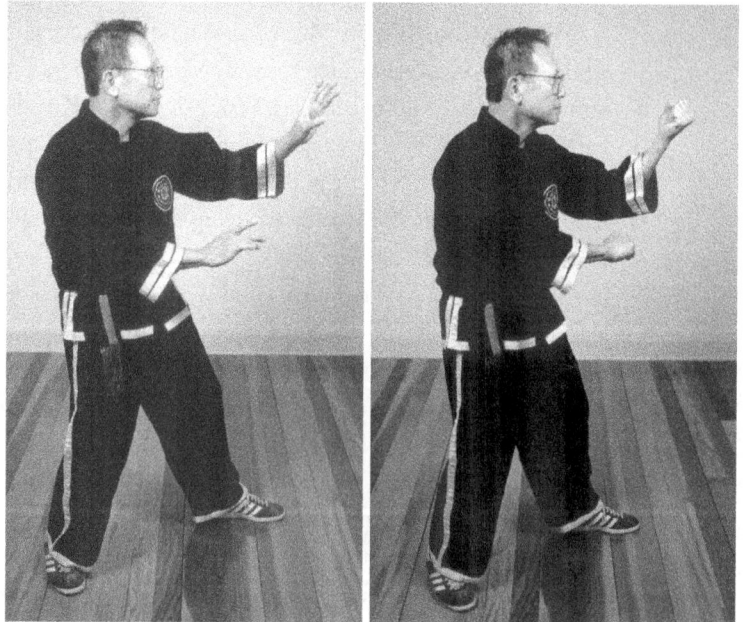

Grandmaster Wai-lun Choi demonstrates the 5 Fists of Hsing-I, from left to right: Piek-Choi (metal), Jin-Choi (water), Beng-Choi (wood), Pao-Choi (fire), and Wang-Choi (earth).

and expense was difficult to manage but he told us sometimes in order to show respect and appreciation money is not important.

After the restaurant Ray and I returned to our hotel to digest a great meal and a lot of information.

The following morning we arrived back at Master Choi's studio for another session before returning home late that afternoon. In this session, we covered new Main Form postures and applications, as well as a lot of discussion and demonstration on body-harmony, speed and power, sensitivity, comparative styles and strategy.

Before we knew it, morning had become afternoon and we invited Master Choi out for one last meal before heading back to the airport. We enjoyed another delightful feast at Li Wing Wa, during which time we arranged to meet with Master Choi once this summer and again in the fall.

Thanks to all our students and friends who contributed to our education fund for making that possible. Wai-lun Choi has continually investigated and questioned the principles and commonly held beliefs in the martial arts for over 40 years in order to reveal their essence — both for himself and for his students.

At one point during our lunch Master Choi joked that he was named Wai because he was always asking why. For Ray and I, that weekend he had a lot more answers than questions.

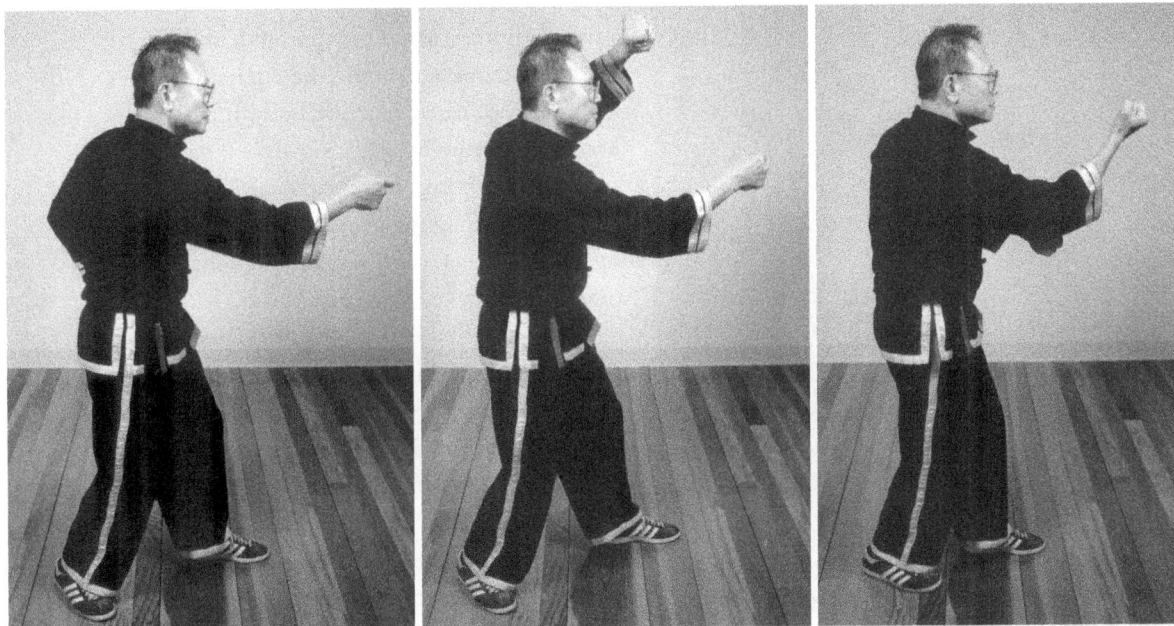

Key Points in the Practice of Liu Ho Pa Fa

Grand Master Wai-lun Choi

(Translated by Anna Yuan, with Eugene Wildman)

The important thing, in my view, is to grasp the experience of the old masters so as to understand what lies behind their development of a successful and reliable training method. It is vital to reveal this, above all, to those who are new to the art, in order that they may avoid the pitfalls of practicing incorrectly. It is something that goes to the core of what is essential in martial arts development. I have a great deal of hands-on experience in Liu Ho Pa Fa, as well as the other internal arts, plus 32 years of practice and contemplation that I would like to share with those who are interested. It is only through careful analysis and sharing that these arts will survive as more than an empty shell.

A martial art is like any other exercise. It is a part of human activity; it pertains to the study of biomechanics and the relation of forces to the structure of the body. It is necessary to employ scientific ideas if we expect to study and teach it effectively. Because it belongs to science rather than opinion or belief, you must submit your practices to the test of proof. You must demonstrate the validity of your claims. For a good idea of the congruence between the thousand-year-old Chinese approach and current scientific research, see for example Philip J. Rasch, *Kinesiology and Applied Anatomy*.

However, a martial art adds another dimension and brings into play something deeper than the physical aspect alone. Liu Ho

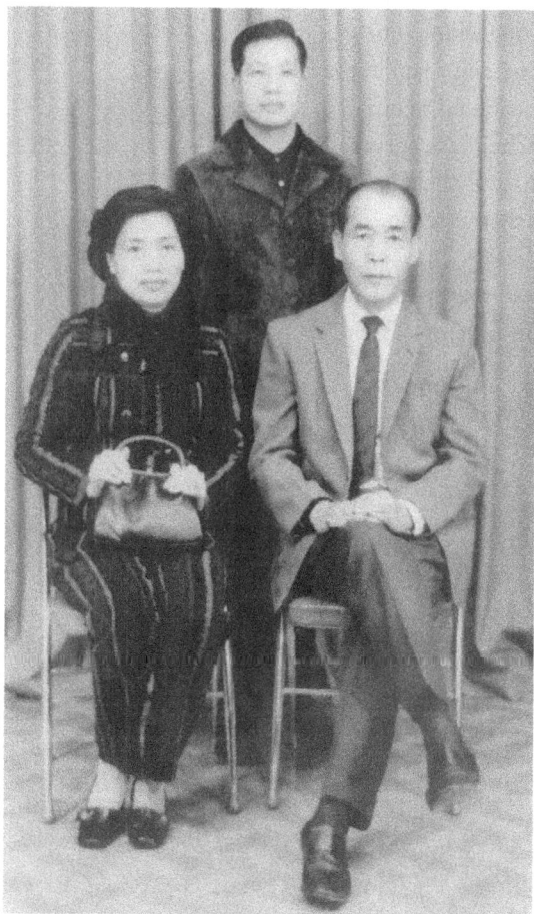

Tenth-generation lineageholder Grandmaster Wai-lun Choi with his teacher, 9th-generation lineageholder Grandmaster Chan Yik-yan and Mrs. Chan in Hong Kong.

Pa Fa not only rests on a foundation of biology, physiology and anatomy, but also the spirit enables its proper performance. Its theory, from every perspective, complies with what is practical and scientifically sound. To develop you must turn away from mysticism and mythology and the belief in secrets that you imagine will transform you. Science and nature are your true teachers; correct training is what will transform you.

Practicing martial arts involves not only factors concerning oneself — physiology, anatomy, psychology and so on — it also requires at least a basic awareness of the principles of physics and the related concepts of leverage, coiling, turning, slanting, triangulation, friction, balance of power, and opposition of forces. If you follow a training program based on such considerations, then your art will improve. You must keep your feet on the ground. By adhering to the instruction of scientific theory, with constant practice and proceeding step by step, you will move to the next level. What follows is intended to add detail to this overview.

1. WHY THE NEED FOR PROOF IN LEARNING MARTIAL ARTS?

With proof your understanding will be clear. Only then can you see through the haze of myths and secrecy that stand in the way of progress. For example, the relation of gravity, air pressure, leverage, physics and so on to the nervous, circulatory and respiratory functions.

2. RELATION OF INTERNAL AND EXTERNAL IN LIU HO PA FA

The full name of the style is Hsing I Liu Ho Pa Fa Ch'uan. "Hsing" represents the outside of things, their form. "I" means the inside, the idea behind the form. The creator of the style saw how animals fight for survival. He noted the form their actions took and grasped the idea behind these actions. What this teaches us is how the spirit and body use the chi and the mind. It shows us how we can use our limbs, bone, muscle to bend and stretch, and how these affect the chi circulation and enable us to improve the body. It relates the chi and the spirit.

You move the way you do because your mind tells you to do something. How the body moves is controlled by the mind. In any situation, first you see, hear, feel. That has to do with the spirit. Spirit is the number one signal. It says *danger*, perhaps, *watch out*.

Mind is the number two signal: it tells you how to do what you do. Where the mind goes, the energy goes too, and then the whole body follows. When the body follows, it is very natural. From this we can see that any movement truly comes from the mind. The mind controls the whole system. The implications of this are considerable. Fake and real, stillness and motion are not separate and have the same root. They all stem from the working of the mind.

3. Relation between Practice and Physiology

The relationship between these two is necessarily close. If you practice wrong you will harm the body; when executing techniques you must be in conformance with physical laws. Each time you move you must search for harmony, for then your breathing will be smooth and regular. The mind must go with the technique.

It is important not to focus on power; you must relax the body. If you do this, the circulation is helped. This cannot be overstressed. The blood is vital. The blood is like a transportation system carrying nutrition and oxygen to make the body strong.

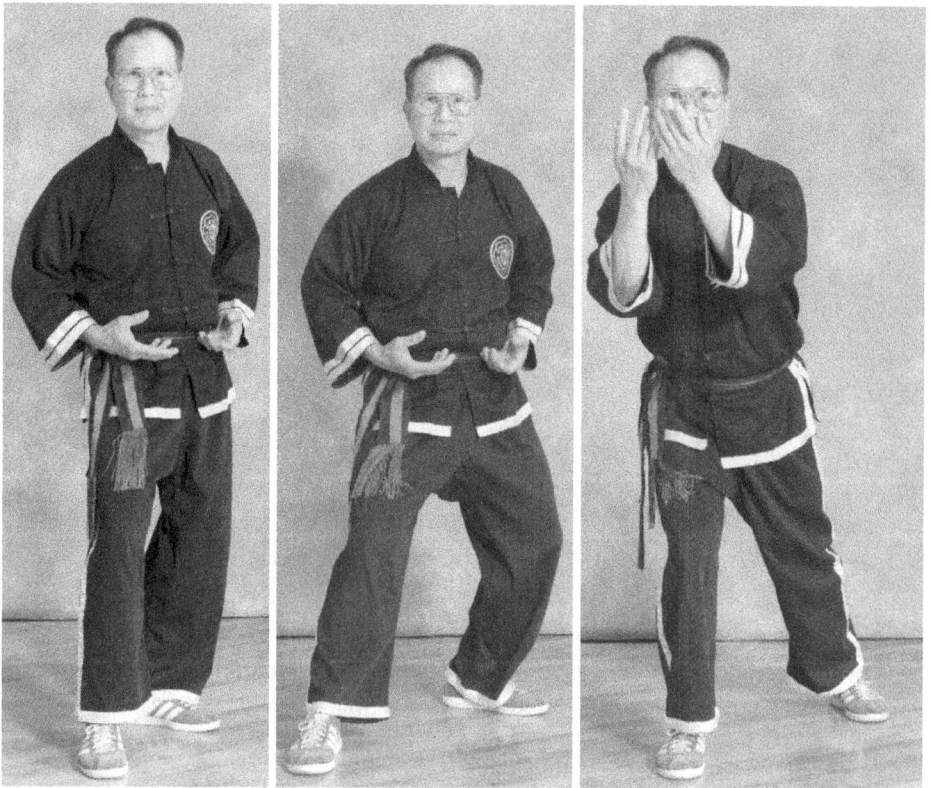

Grandmaster Wai-lun Choi demonstrates four movements of the Dragon posture from the Liu Ho Pa Fa 12 Animals set. Notice the animal fighting spirit projecting from Sifu Choi's eyes.

4. Relation of Breathing System to Tensing and Relaxing

Whether moving or still, relaxation is crucial. You need to relax the whole body in order to breathe normally. Only then can your circulation be good. If you are nervous, or if you force the power, you will tense your muscles, especially around the chest, and the breathing will be unnatural.

5. Relation between Movement and Breathing

When you are practicing, every movement must have harmony. The reason is because there are three parts to the whole body: the body proper, the hands, the feet. Suppose if you punched the hands went first, then the feet, then the body followed. This would violate what the Classics say: one thing moves, everything moves. But why do they say that?

The reason is because it has a direct connection to breathing. One technique done incorrectly, as above, will require three breaths and make the breathing fast. This is why the old masters insisted if one thing moves, everything must move. The correct way is body-hand-foot together. In other words, one breath, inhale or exhale, one energy. If you don't follow the Classics there will be no oxygen and thus no energy.

Try an experiment. First punch to experience how you breathe; then move your foot after that and you will see for yourself what the old masters found. I have no doubt it took much time and much real, even painful experience to come up with this one-thing-moves-all-things-move theory, and I deeply admire their analytical intelligence.

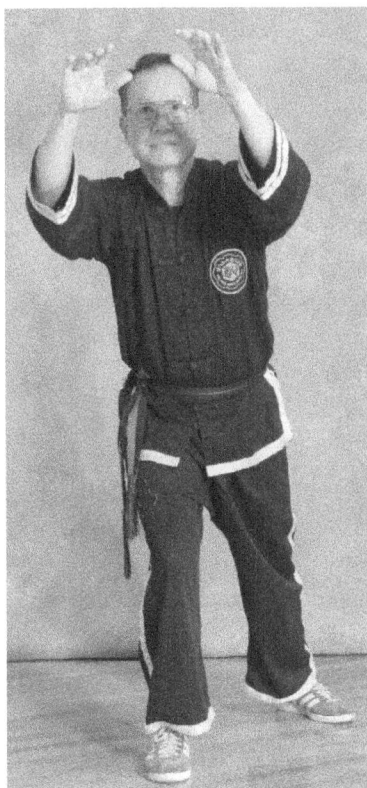

6. Relation of Physics to Bones and Joint Function

The old masters created techniques, all of which follow physics and physiology. Therefore, when practicing pay attention in every technique that the shoulder and elbow are down, the chest rounded and so on. Every movement must follow correct principles in order to have a complete and effective technique. The bones allow us to use leverage; the joints may be compared to a switch that enables us to change the angle and thus the leverage.

7. The relation of leverage to correct practice

Optimal performance comes from observing correct principles. In sparring, for instance, you must always pay attention to leverage. Only then can you reach a natural, relaxed state, save energy and save power. As the T'ai-Chi Classics say, "Use four ounces to defeat a thousand pounds." Or take the case of Japanese judo. In both instances what is involved is leverage. In a real-world situation, everyone's body type is different. But if you follow leverage theory, the weak can defeat the strong, the small can overcome the large.

8. Relation of psychology to performance

Cultivation of a strong, tough mind can change the state of a person. If the body is not healthy, you cannot have a good psychological state, to say nothing of high aspirations. And even if you do have good ideas, if you lack energy you will not be able to carry them out. Let some external factor get in your way and you will lose your confidence and be unable to move forward.

A person who does martial arts, though, not only should have a healthy body, he should have confidence in his daily affairs. Presented with difficulties, he can use his energy and strength of mind to deal with the problem. He will have the courage to face it. If your art is at a high level, you necessarily have energy and courage; with courage your skill automatically is at a higher level.

This higher level skill that appears alongside courage is not only in regard to the body. More important is how it cultivates the spirit. The martial arts use psychology from beginning to end in their training. You must concentrate your spirit in your daily practice. If you do, you will not have any fear. If you have no fear, in a fighting situation your mind will be very strong. It is something that shows up in daily practice: in concentration, in the absence of fear, in the readiness to act. These are three essential qualities.

Many years ago on television I saw an American Olympic high jumper. Before he jumped he concentrated his spirit, judging how many steps he would need before he made his jump. He used his mind in order to succeed. When you do that, you enter the psychological state that is necessary for achieving success.

The proper state not only allows you to have confidence physically, but when you have difficulties or must confront an opponent, you will always maintain a clear mind and believe that you can win. In such a state, you will be able to react immediately and easily.

9. Relation of Mind to Nervous System Function

Any exercise is controlled by the nervous system. Proper neural functioning is what allows the muscles to stretch and contract. The bones have to do with leverage; the joints enable us to change leverage, as noted, while the muscles produce movement and delivery of power. It is how all activity shows up in the body. From this we can see clearly the critical role the nervous system, plays in controlling bodily activity. But the nervous system, from beginning to end, is influenced by the spirit and the mind. The mind is the ruler of the power.

Why do the Classics insist on that? If you talk about Hsing I, that is form-idea, you are emphasizing mind. Liu Ho Pa Fa uses mind in the name to point to its cruciality. In martial arts the mind is of central importance. A skilled painter, for instance, must have a detailed image in his mind in order to be able to transfer it to paper. It is the same in martial arts. If you separate the mind from the power, then you are unable to bring it to bear.

The whole art presupposes a very high level of unification of the spirit and the body. If you don't have the body to show the form, the mind is only an image, an idea. If you don't have the mind, you have a blind form. You cannot have one without the other. No real fighter would dare to use a form alone, or merely imaginary power, against the muscle and bone and sinew of an actual flesh-and-blood adversary.

Contributor's Note: Wai-lun Choi is the designated grandmaster of the Liu Ho Pa Fa style. In 1971 he was the All-Southeast Asia full-contact champion. He is also an expert in T'ai-Chi, Hsing-I, Pa Kua, Lama, Thai boxing, and more. He has served as Hsing-I advisor of the U.S. Kuo Shu Association.

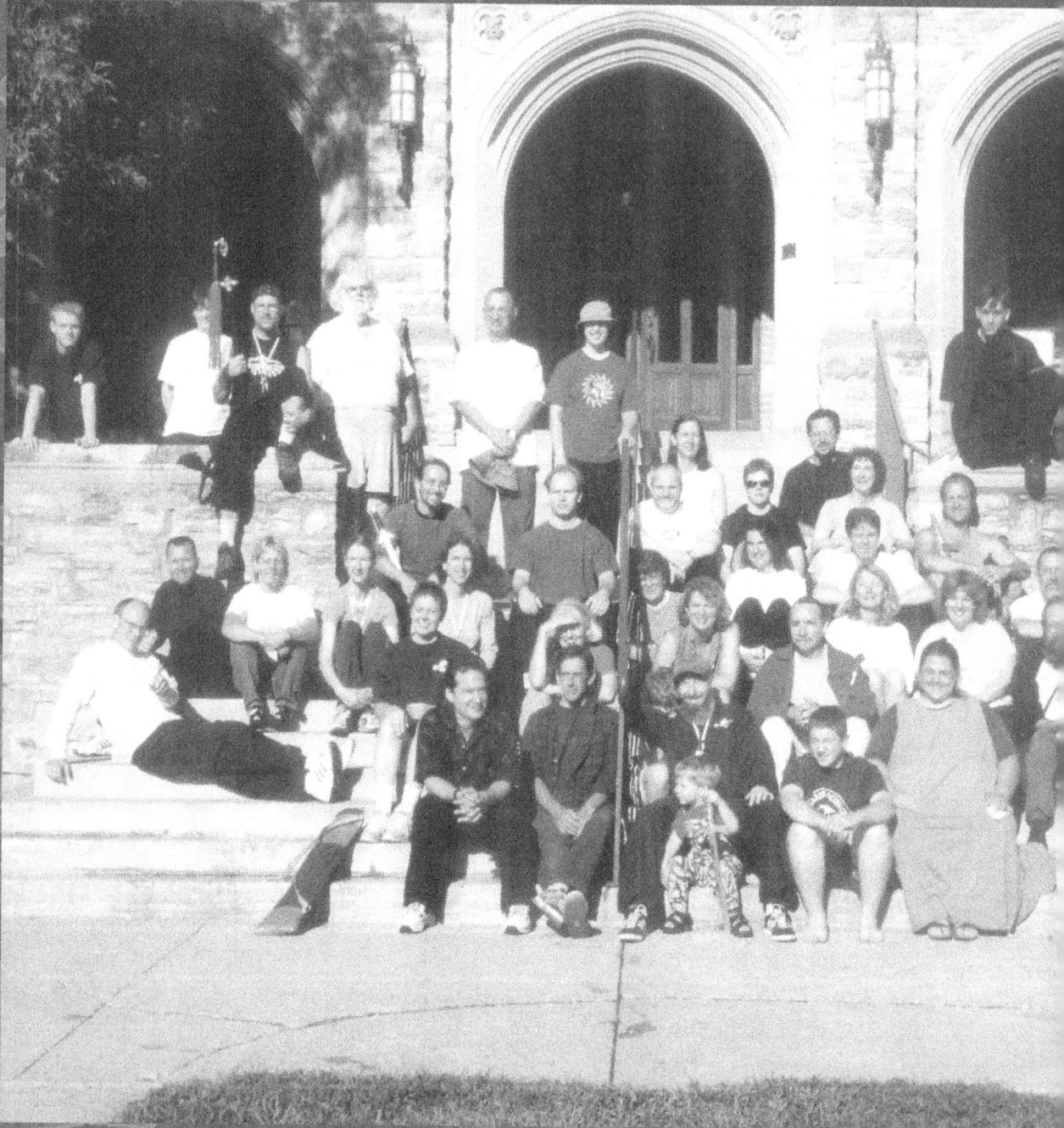

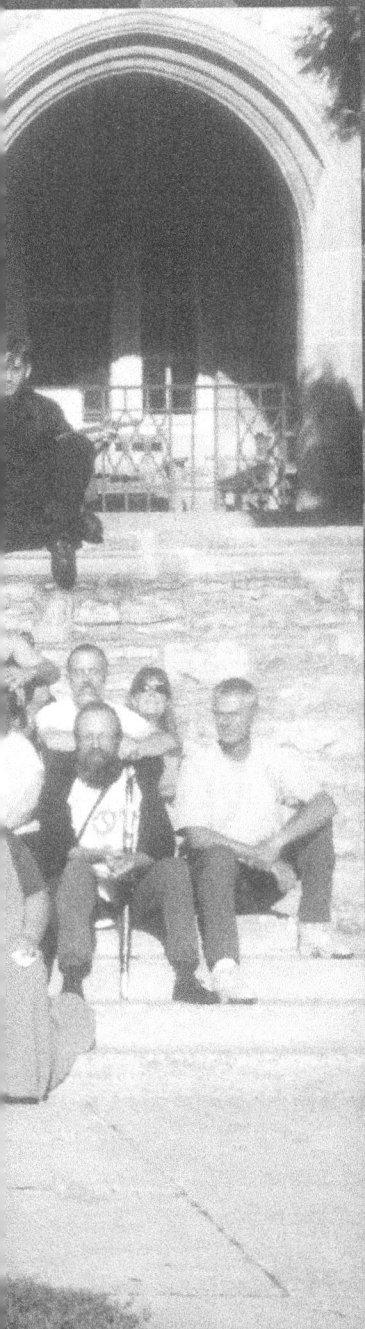

FUTURE

曙 ☯ 光

In February 1989, Ray and Paul began initiating the seventh generation of lineage-holders. In this section, several of them and their fellow students share their thoughts, through essay, poetry and a fantastic cake recipe, on the role T'ai-Chi plays in their lives.

Opposite page: The 3rd Annual Twin Cities T'ai Chi Ch'uan Retreat in Faribault, Minnesota (2001).

First Class:
December 23, 1993

Elyse Duffy, 7th-generation lineageholder, 2002

Rushing. Christmas shopping. Wrapping, cards, groceries. Crowded stores. Maniac drivers. University Avenue choked with them.

There's that T'ai-Chi place. Who told me? Tom. Mary's friend. Dinner party. Said it was good.

Christ! That idiot nearly hit me! Done with this. Stop. Get a brochure.

Cold, concrete warehouse turned cheap artist rentals. Hand-written signs, like breadcrumbs, point the way down dusty halls. Not sure about this.

Around the corner, half a dozen people — there's Tom — waiting outside a locked door.

Late instructor. Not impressed.

No literature. Less impressed.

About to leave when he shows up. No hurry, all smiles. Ask if I can watch. Just five minutes.

No, he says. Not surprised. Instead, take the class. No charge.

Shocked. Is he joking? Is this a game? Some crazy-wisdom T'ai-Chi test?

He seems serious. Very strange. Never happen in ballet. Two months tuition, in advance. Out of town visitors show a union card. Observation not allowed. Period.

Unsure, I hesitate. But he's convincing. His name is Ray.

暉 ☯ 光

Small class, eight or ten people. All women, except for Tom. And Ray. First a warm-up — pretty easy. Then some Qigong. I've heard of it — traditional form of healing. But I don't know what it has to do with T'ai-Chi. Simple arm movements coordinated with the breath. I like it. It's relaxing.

Then we do the "form." I follow along as best I can. The movements aren't that complex, but still I struggle to keep up. At least they're slow, which helps.

It's nearly silent; the only sounds the protest of a creaky board or squeak of a damp tennis shoe.

I try to keep my eyes on Ray, even when suddenly we turn and my back is to him — or should be. He is fluid. Controlled. Long legs, strong and flexible. But nothing showy.

I try to feel what the movement feels like to him. Inside his body. To transfer it into mine. Too much. I lose my place and stumble to catch up.

I watch the others when I can't contort to see Ray. They all seem to know what they're doing. There's one woman in particular who astounds me. She must be close to mom's age. But so vital. So strong. So…certain. Are these the effects of T'ai-Chi? Or is she just an exceptional woman?

It takes a long time, longer than I expected. Twenty or thirty minutes. Then everyone stops, silent, frozen for a few seconds. I'm not tired or spent, but I know I've done something. My legs tingle.

The spell breaks and they all just wander off. No closure. No applause. No révérence. Strange place.

I like it.

暉 ☯ 光

In the dressing room, I replay the class. It will always be like this: Follow along, get what you can, stumble, fall, try again. Like ballet.

I have a sheet that has all the "postures" listed. Prosaic names like "Fair Lady Weaves at the Shuttles" and "Carry Tiger, Return to Mountain." There are 150 all told, but some of them repeat.

Maybe only 100 to learn — ever. Always the same order, no variations. Everything's to one side — nothing gets reversed. Easier than ballet. Two, maybe three months, and I should have it down.

But then what? If you just do the same thing over and over, where's the challenge? Hmmph. Guess I'll worry about that later.

I write a check for one month's tuition: $50.00 for unlimited classes (How do these people make a living?), but Ray has disappeared. Come late, leave early. Nice schedule.

The woman I admired in class walks by and I stop her. She takes my check and tosses it on the cluttered desk. Whatever. With luck he'll find it before the next one's due. Not my problem.

Grab my coat. I have to get to Snyder's, the co-op, gotta call…

She stops me — the woman with the check.

Where are you going?

Grocery store for starters, I think. Then Paper Warehouse, then…

Ray wants me to work with you.

Work with me? What the hell does that mean?

曙 ☯ 光

Her name is Joanne and she takes me to one corner of the studio, by a small altar I haven't noticed before. I'm only vaguely aware that Ray teaches the rest of the class across the room.

Joanne starts with Qigong. Breathing in, breathing out, she shows me the first half-dozen movements. They were simple before, but now I can begin to analyze, memorize.

Then we dive into the "first section." Step-by-step, count-by-count, Joanne breaks down the postures. I'm surprised by the counting. Each posture has two, four, or six counts, and hearing them helps me learn the movements.

Something familiar to anchor to. I wonder why they didn't count earlier, when we did the whole form. Everyone must count in their heads.

Joanne recites the names: Ward Off Left, Roll Back, Press, Push, Single Whip. But just like plié, tendu, and dégagé, I don't try to remember them. The names will come later, with repetition. For now, the movement is all I want.

She shows me tiny details, but just as I begin to absorb one movement, she moves on to the next. I don't take it all in — it's unusual movement for me: understated and small. I want to go back to the beginning, now that my eyes can see the logic. Repeat over and over. But we keep moving forward, another posture, another posture. My mind goes into overload.

Ray Hayward demonstrates Bend the Bow to Shoot the Tiger.

I start to panic, tension rising in my stomach and flowing upward. I can't remember what we just did. I need to remember the sequence. It's key. What comes next? What comes next?? To be seen, to earn a correction, to get a role, you have to know sequence. I won't remember all this!

Joanne says to breathe into my abdomen and I pull myself back from ballet flashbacks and see the room anew. The breathing is familiar from meditation. I let my belly expand and I relax. Maybe there aren't any roles in T'ai-Chi.

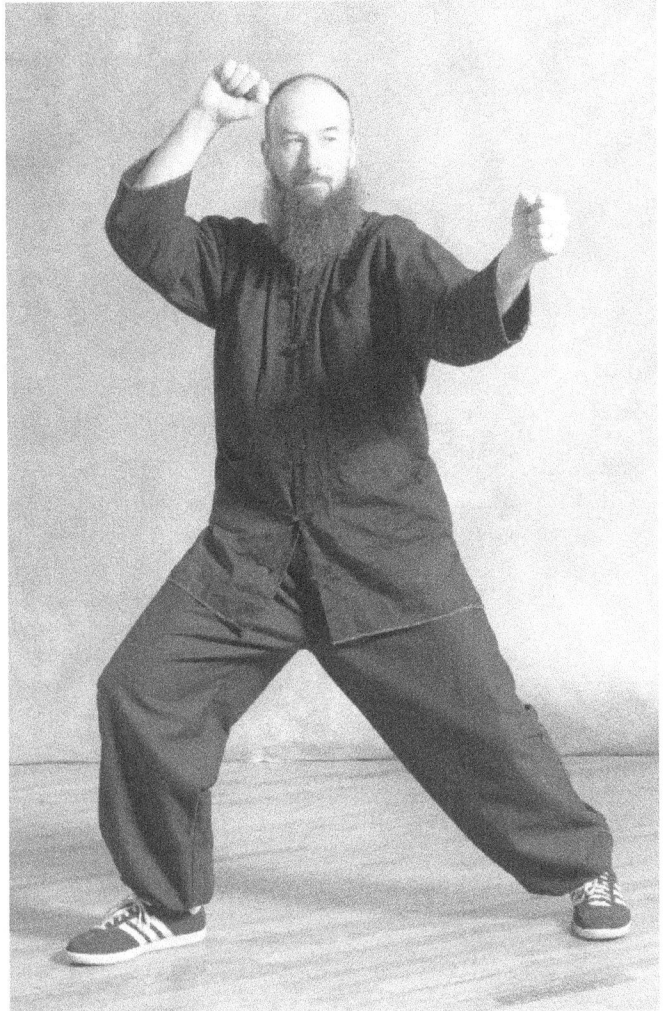

And then we're done. It takes a few seconds for me to re-orient. It's been over an hour. An hour! I'm shell-shocked.

In ballet, coaching is reserved for soloists and principals. But here, I walk in the door and they give it away. Free. I've been here almost two hours, and just had an hour of one-on-one instruction. I can't quite process that.

I'm so amazed I almost forget to thank Joanne. She is gracious and seems to think nothing of it.

Suddenly I remember I have to get to the bank before the drive-up closes. I grab my coat and look for Ray, but this time he's really gone.

I fly down the stairs, not ready to face the traffic on University.

But there's the cat food to pick up,

the co-op before it's too busy,

call the folks,

vacuum,

laundry,

wrapping...

All I Really Need To Know I Learned In Beginner's Class

Dan Nave, 7th-generation lineageholder, 2002

A friend once confided that he found it difficult to teach T'ai-Chi. There seemed to be little that he could find to say about it other than to experience it. In fact, during the first lesson he told students pretty much everything he thought they needed to know. His advice was, "No matter what technique you are doing, relax and sink."

Relaxation seems like a simple notion — unless you don't do it.

Physically, the idea is to use those muscles that are necessary to sustain a particular posture or movement and to relax those which are not necessary. After all, you don't need to clench your jaw in order to stand upright. Any movement involving extension does not need the muscles involved in contraction, so they should be relaxed. Using extraneous muscles in an action impedes that action and wastes a lot of energy.

Being aware of the experience of physical relaxation leads one to the idea of structure. An inefficient body structure will require many more

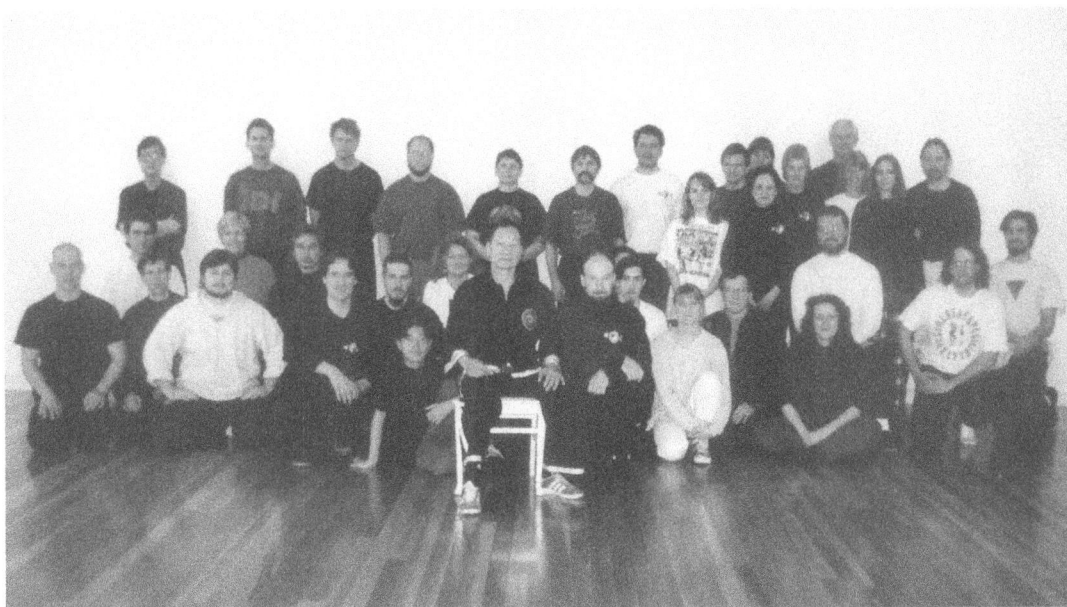

Grandmaster Wai-lun Choi's first seminar at Twin Cities T'ai Chi Ch'uan in 1995.

muscles at a higher degree of effort to sustain it, reducing relaxation. The awareness and practice of relaxation will reveal this.

Relaxation also applies to the mind and mental process. Concentration involves not so much effort as it does getting rid of those mental processes that distract. Concentration involves mental relaxation. Thoughts such as, "Why did they make me stand in the middle of the group — I must look like an idiot" leave very little mental process left to experience T'ai-Chi. As in the physical, mental structures should be flexible and fluid. Rigidity of thinking restricts possibility, restricts creativity, and restricts the wider experience of reality.

Relaxation on a more subtle level might be applied to dogma, beliefs and conditioning. Everyone carries a lot of extra "baggage" of this sort with them. Find out what is extraneous and relax your grip on it. Let it fall away.

The concept of "sink" is more obscure, and I would hesitate to define it. It is a feeling that comes through practice. After relaxation one may find dissipation or centeredness. To sink is to find the center, to find a root, physically, mentally or spiritually.

Nevertheless, the Tao, as experienced through T'ai-Chi, is a path to be walked not terms to be explained.

So, as Master Po might have said, "Relax and sink, Grasshopper, and by the way, don't forget to experience."

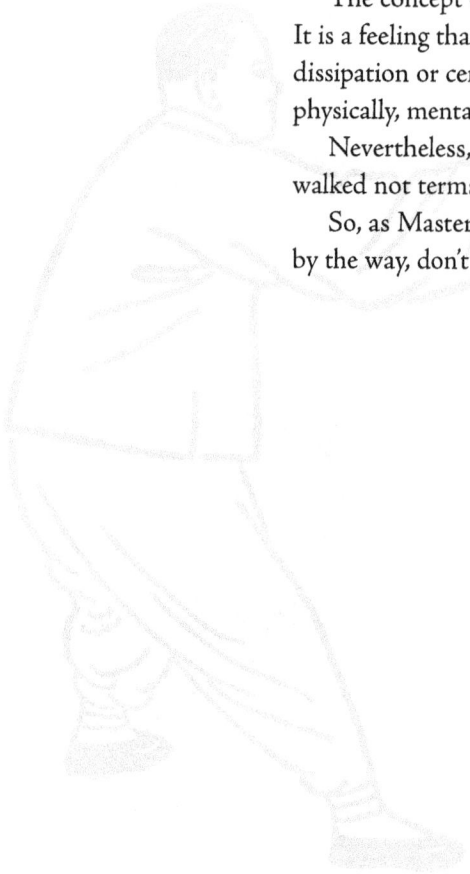

GROWTH

SALLY POLK, 7TH-GENERATION LINEAGEHOLDER, 2002

Twin Cities T'ai-Chi Ch'uan's 10-year anniversary of teaching and practicing the Yang-style T'ai-Chi Ch'uan in our beautiful studio is indeed a cause for celebration. After several previous moves, we found our current, most suitable and attractive studio in 1992, and thanks to Joanne and Phil, were able to put in the good wooden floor.

In this flow of time, we've witnessed growth in number and in skills of our studio members, and I continue to experience increasing respect and gratitude for the many excellences of instruction, interpretation and friendship that our leaders, Ray and Paul, share with us.

I met Master Liang only twice, both at studio demonstrations for him, once in our studio down University Avenue and once in our current Twin Cities T'ai-Chi Ch'uan studio. I've known Master Liang most through stories told by Ray and Paul, by their teaching and through Master Liang's book.

My own T'ai-Chi Ch'uan journey began in the fall of 1982, studying first with Jonah Friedman, then Ray, Jonah, Paul and Joanne. I continue to grow in appreciation of the benefits of T'ai-Chi Ch'uan for physical and mental health, strength, balance, meditation and well-being, as well as each posture's applications for self-defense. I appreciate the relaxed atmosphere in our studio, created by Ray and Paul, the feeling of openness and acceptance of many different kinds of people who learn in many different ways.

I admire Ray's and Paul's desire for and practice of new forms, their ongoing quest for new knowledge, interpretation, integration and application, their growing skills in teaching. We are fortunate to have them as our most excellent teachers, and fortunate that Master T.T. Liang, as part of the Yang family tradition, was their teacher, and more, and also ours.

We each seem to need to learn patience and the willingness to commit time to practice each movement 100 x 100 times — and more.

I've been reading Ray's book, *Lessons with Master T.T. Liang* (2000), and have chosen a few quotes that have particular resonance for me.

This is whole life business, this T'ai-Chi. If you get addicted to it, you cannot get rid of it. (p. 23)

T'ai-Chi for self-defense is whole life business. It takes practicing year after year to get anything. Even 10 years is only a short time to practice. (p. 60)

Don't think of the future or the past, only the present. (p. 82)

You must learn to yield. That way, in times of emergency, you will know how to deal with people. (p. 83)

If you practice T'ai-Chi for a long time it should change your temperament. (p. 85)

I'm teaching you to yield. I try to intimidate you. If you laugh, you win. If you get angry, I win. (p. 86)

Everything is different. Everything changes, so adapt to the circumstances. (p. 89)

When a teacher wants to hand down his art, he must find out if his student is really good. Otherwise, the teacher's time and effort are wasted. I want my students to get better than I am. If they aren't better, that means my art is terrible — cannot be handed down to anybody. This exercise, T'ai-Chi, is for everybody, whole-world exercise. (p. 88)

I'm grateful to Master T.T. Liang — the vibrations of his teaching and who he was will continue to echo. And I'm especially grateful to Ray and Paul during this tenth year in our current Twin Cities T'ai-Chi Ch'uan studio for all they continue to do and are for all our students, and for me.

A Gift of Clouds

Linda Hermanson, 7th-generation lineageholder, 2002

It was 1984 when Rosemary, Barbara, Joan and I started T'ai-Chi lessons with Jonah Friedman as our instructor. Jonah was a student of Master T.T. Liang, so not much later that year, we started traveling to St. Cloud every other Saturday to study with T.T. himself. Being in his 80s at the time didn't stop him from having way more energy than us and having a hilarious sense of humor.

One of my favorite memories was the day we began to learn the Wave Hands in Clouds postures. As usual, it was a lot of fun as well as work, and on the ride home the full effect of the lesson was realized. I saw the clouds and the sky in a completely new way. They had never before seemed so beautiful and alive. I knew I had experienced something extraordinary that was transmitted by Master Liang through T'ai-Chi. It was such a gift.

Now, many years later, as I have learned and forgotten much about the forms, T'ai-Chi still sustains me and adds much to my life. I am deeply grateful to Ray Hayward and Paul Abdella, long-time students and disciples of Master Liang's, for providing the expertise, space and love of T'ai-Chi so that it is available to so many and at such a high level.

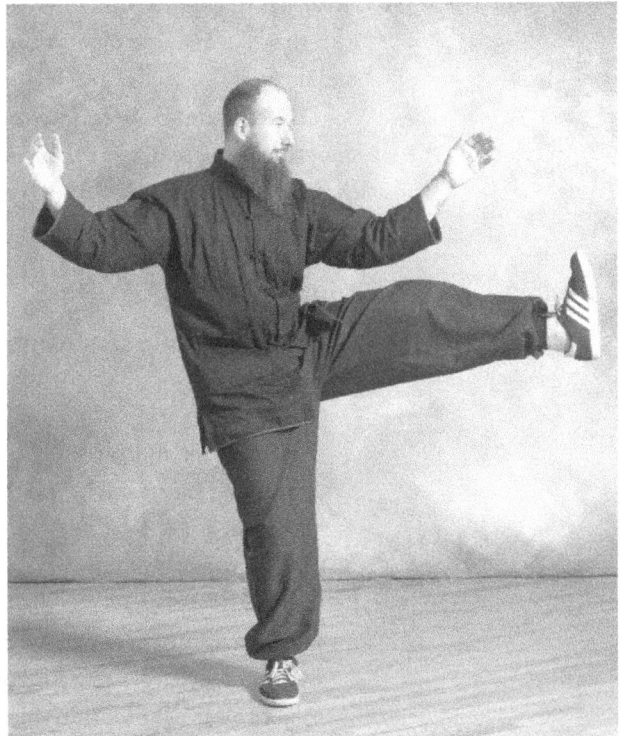

Ray Hayward demonstrates Kick Upward with the Left Foot.

Chocolate Oblivion Truffle Torte

Woody Wolston, 7th-generation lineageholder, 2002

From Rose Levy Beranbaum's **The Cake Bible**, *1988*

Editor's note: Woody bakes fantastic cakes for birthdays and other special occasions at the studio. This one is the most popular and the most decadent.

This is the cake most requested of me by T'ai-Chi studio members and broomball players' wives. Although simple to make, it looks unusual as well as elegant. It transports well. I have hauled this hundreds of miles in coolers, with the cake maintaining its flavor and shape, to see it evaporate with smiling faces.

This cake can be best described as a baked mousse — a very rich and smooth chocolate dessert that melts in your mouth. You bake it like a cheesecake. (WARNING: Forget the calorie count!)

Enjoy!

Ingredients

Have all ingredients at room temperature.

Ingredients	Volume	Weight
bittersweet chocolate	22 ounces	22 ounces
unsalted butter	22 ounces	22 tablespoons
large eggs (7-8)	1 ⅔ cups	14.2 ounces

Equipment

+ 9-inch springform pan for cake
+ 10-inch or larger pan for cooking water bath
+ large glass or microwavable bowl for melting chocolate
+ 2-qt. bowl for the eggs
+ large bowl for combining the chocolate and eggs

Recipe

1. Preheat oven to 425 degrees F.

2. Fill with 1 inch of water a 10-inch or larger pan or cake pan for making a water bath. Heat water to a simmer on the stove.

3. Prepare a 9" springform pan:
   + Cut a 9" wax paper round
   + Butter the bottom and sides of the pan, put round on bottom, and butter the round
   + Wrap the outside with a double layer of heavy-duty foil to prevent seepage in the water bath

4. Chop the chocolate into small pieces.

5. Melt the chocolate and butter together in either the top of a double boiler over simmering water OR in a glass bowl placed in the microwave. If using microwave, set at high power, stirring every 20 seconds. Remove from heat when almost melted and stir to complete melting. Let stand at room temperature

6. Prepare the eggs. Put eggs in a large bowl. Hold the bowl over the water bath pan to heat up the eggs. Stir and break the egg yolks until the eggs are warm to touch with no cooked whites.

7. Remove the eggs from heat and beat until triple in volume and forming soft peaks when raised with a whisk beater in a standing mixer. OR Beat over the heated water bath with a hand mixer until triple in volume (this takes about 5 minutes).

8. Pour the melted chocolate and butter into a large bowl. Fold half of the whipped eggs into the chocolate and butter using a metal whisk or large rubber spatula until almost incorporated. Fold in the rest of the eggs until just blended and showing no streaks. Finish with a rubber spatula, scraping the bottom heavier mixture up to incorporate.

9. Pour and smooth the mixture into the springform pan.

10. Bake the cake. Place the water bath pan on the middle rack of the oven. Place the springform pan in the water bath. It will be floating. Bake for 5 minutes. Cover loosely with a piece of metal foil and bake 10 more minutes.

11. Cool the cake. Remove from oven and place on a cooling rack. Cake will look soft in the middle. Cool for at least 45 minutes. Cover with plastic wrap and refrigerate for at least 3 hours.

12. Remove the cake from the springform pan. Rub the sides of the pan with a very hot, dampened towel to melt the sides of the cake a little. (You can also heat up a knife blade and run it on the outside of the cake.) Release and remove the springform pan's side.

13. Put a piece of wax paper on top of the cake, then a plate or cookie sheet, and invert. Reheat the damp towel and the rub the bottom of the springform pan to warm it. Use a knife to pry the bottom away from the cake and wax paper liner. Peel off the wax paper liner. Re-invert the cake onto a serving plate or cake carrier bottom.

To cut the cake: Heat up a knife blade and cut the cake and pull through. Wipe off the blade if it gets too much chocolate on it. A slice of an inch wide is plenty.

Specifications

+ Cake will serve 16 to 18.

+ Bring to room temperature for best flavor and texture.

+ Storage: 6 hours at room temperature. Refrigerated for 2 weeks. Cake cannot be frozen.

+ Time: 45 minutes to prep, 15 minutes to bake, 45 minutes cooling rack, 3 hours to refrigerate.

Additions

Blend 2 to 3 tablespoons of your favorite espresso or liqueur into the melted chocolate.

Adornments

Sweetened whipped cream by itself or with liqueur flavoring

A white chocolate (6 ounces) and cream (1.5 ounces) glaze. (Melt in microwave. Cool to room temperature. Pour and spread on top of cake.)

Raspberry sauce without seeds

What a Way to Enjoy Living for the Rest of Your Life!

Woody Wolston, 7th-generation lineageholder, 2002

I'm amazed by the doors that have been opened by practicing T'ai-Chi and being a member of this studio.

My interest in T'ai-Chi was simply a challenge to learn a 150-posture form, one that a few black belts had learned at the karate club I used to attend. (I stopped attending due to some lower back injuries resulting in me not being able to kick above the waist. I was not the most popular person to spar.) I had enjoyed doing the 15- to 35-posture karate forms.

I have to thank Jon Engstrom twice. After I learned the first section of the form at the St. Paul Jewish Community Center, he convinced me to come to the studio. Then he and Ray let me take over teaching at the JCC, for the last five years.

Remember that first class? "Hi, glad you could come." "Here is the schedule." "Oh don't worry, we start at 6:10." You were welcomed and given a summary of the class routine. Then you spotted the head instructor sitting on his chair and talking to a group of students. Maybe some "shop talk" for you to eavesdrop in on. But no, he was telling a funny story and everyone was laughing.

Another person, who you figured must be an instructor judging by the two students who beelined for him, walked into the studio. He started conversing. You were amazed by his eyes and facial expressions that maximized the story that he had just told.

At 6:10, class commenced with the stretches and standing meditation. "Am I doing this right?" you asked yourself as you wondered when the T'ai-Chi was going to start. You were then treated like someone very special, given personal instruction, and at the end of the form — although a bit embarrassed from all those wrong turns — you were smiling from ear to ear. What a rush!

Then with following visits to the studio, you not only were able to have Ray and Paul let their knowledge rush into you on T'ai-Chi (and the other styles offered) at the speed you wanted to assimilate it, but you were now part of a community. A community of positive-minded people willing to: share knowledge, offer their services, give great referrals, go out for coffee, and give back to the studio. You kept practicing and your health, posture, and physical health kept improving.

You then got to attend summer retreats. You saw the community come through again in jam sessions, bridge marathons, ping-pong and badminton wars, and just plain fun times. And you found that if you need help beyond the studio, there is a bulletin board plastered with business cards. "I see this chiropractor." "This is a really good tea blend for a sore throat." "Rolfing helps to align your body's connective tissue."

Hopefully, you all have a significant other who can enjoy the changes in you. Although my wife, Susan, is having a harder time finding a place to tickle me, she is happy to see me not the hyper ping-pong ball of years before. And she enjoys her piece of cake, too.

We all have many thanks for the discovering of this vibrant studio rooted in T.T Liang's knowledge, broadened by Ray's and Paul's searches for knowledge from many great masters, and their own revelations. It's a growing studio due to its excellent overseeing board of directors, the heart of Joanne Von Blon, and the ambassadors that we all are in spreading the news.

I recently ran into a friend at a restaurant I had not seen for four years. He remarked, "Woody, you look younger." I guess we are all on the right path.

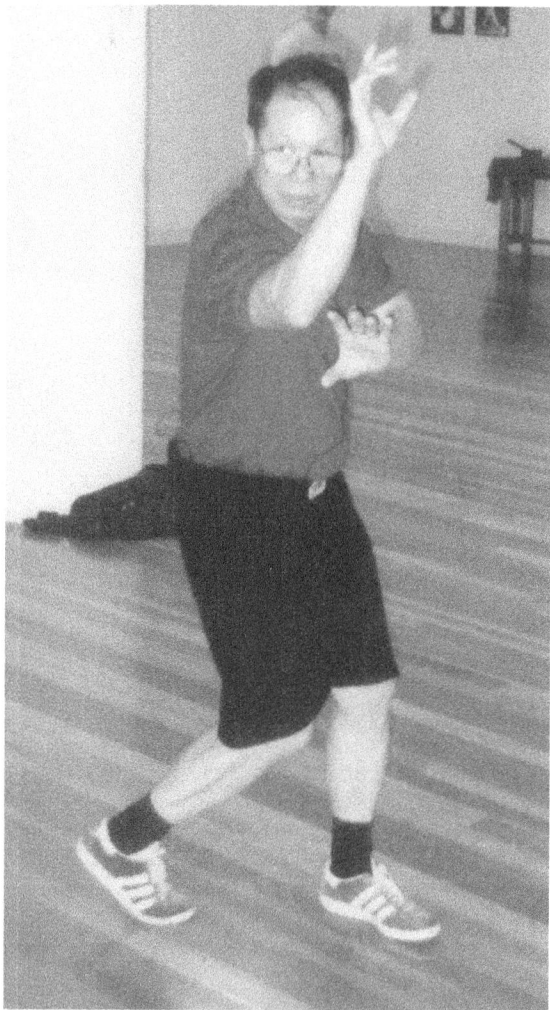

Grandmaster Choi "Running the Circle" in a Pa Kua seminar.

READING BETWEEN THE LINES

LaVonne Bunt, 2001

Ray,
Congratulations, as you celebrate 25 years of T'ai-Chi. I thank you for your
friendship and all the wisdom you have so generously shared. I share with you
a few humble words of a beginner in this quest toward mastery.

As I have practiced T'ai-Chi over these past three years, I have learned lessons on many levels. T'ai-Chi is a study in contrasts amidst an utter simplicity of movement. Mastering the fluid harmony of breath, posture and quiet mind will be a lifelong study. For me, levels of understanding find their center beyond the martial application of each movement.

T'ai-Chi is an art of reading between the lines. It is a study of complementary opposites: strength in softness, power emanating from yielding. It is a gentle art that draws on an inner core strength each of us holds deep within our being. For some of us that strength gets buried deep enough to appear inaccessible. But as it surfaces for even the briefest of moments, everything changes. It is an insight that goes deeper than cliché or metaphor.

Time, energy, and enduring patience are pieces of my learning process. (As a realist, I readily admit that frustration with the process is also instructive.) Absorbing with understanding the subtle details among the broad strokes of this art comes much later. I am only beginning to scratch the surface of a whole discipline and way of seeing from a

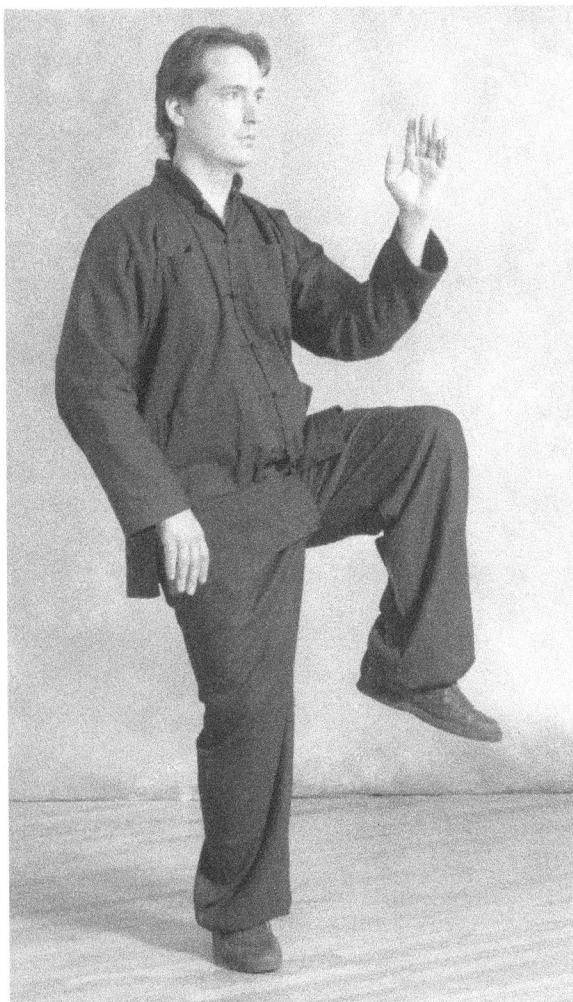

Paul Abdella demonstrates Golden Rooster Standing on One Leg (left).

T'ai-Chi perspective. The practice, even with those disarming attempts to learn a new form, changes me. As I go deeper, the nuances emerge level by level, each expanding on a previous moment of insight.

The T'ai-Chi Classics, Ray, Paul, and Master Liang's wisdom each put those precious pieces of the puzzle in plain sight long before I see to understand. Practice and application do shed light on those elusive strands that connect a formidable "string of pearls" that the Classics describe.

As I hear echoes to relax and sink into a posture with a quiet mind, I become aware in my own practice of how significant a role the mind plays. Without focused intent, the process becomes mechanical and fragmented. I am not sure when or how that piece opened up. How a quiet mind changes the whole dynamic is part of the puzzle. It directs and gives context to the whole discipline. It offers a sense of depth in understanding how my own center is aligned and how I read the line of a partner's movement.

While sequence and technique without doubt are critically important, the mind intent is the dimension that offers a key to going deeper in my practice. For me it is the most challenging aspect to unravel. In my own practice it is a chasm not yet crossed. There are moments in which I touch the shadows of that focused tranquillity. As I place trust in my teachers and fellow students, and ultimately in my own being, I hope to expand upon that learning. Working with brilliant teachers and fellow students illuminates dimensions of this experience in ways that continue to amaze me. It is a work in progress. There is much to be learned reading between the lines.

Energy Follows Thought

James Whitney, 7th-generation lineageholder, 2002

Taoist arts are multifaceted. Regular practice yields many benefits such as vibrant health, the ability to defend oneself against physical attack, and the rather ephemeral promise of enlightenment. (It is assumed that those seeking enlightenment are not already enlightened; few seek what they currently possess.)

Much care is given to students to ensure that they develop a solid physical foundation, or a root. It is from a strong root that effective techniques proceed and that good health is restored and maintained. It is also from this root that the quest for enlightenment grows. This may prove more difficult. People live in a world of conditioning that is reinforced daily. Who can honestly say that most, if not all, definitions regarding the self, the root, are not those imposed by others?

Based upon my own practice, I have some ideas that may prove helpful in discovering one's own essence, free from the opinions of others, as well as a method to strengthen this spiritual root so that one may attain that to which one aspires.

First of all, one should assume that one is totally free, without limit or obligation. Then one needs to decide what one would be in such a state. This may take some time, but it is worth the effort. At first, it is likely that one will seek to fulfill one's conditioning. Assume you are alone and that you create the people and situations in your life. After some time, the truth will be uncovered — the true desire, the cherished hope, the Holy Grail. At this point, there is a need to choose a method, or a path to reach the goal.

As I said, the Taoist arts provide such a path. In T'ai-Chi, one is advised to relax and sink. This advice also applies to the self. One acknowledges one's nature and what it desires and allows it to manifest. This is to "do without doing." One intends that the physical practice of T'ai-Chi issues from the root of the spiritual center.

Don Juan told Carlos Castaneda that the tonal, or the external, world was a manifestation of the nagual, the spirit world. Hence, energy expressed physically is the result of intent based upon the root. Chi (energy) follows yi (intent).

With continued practice, one may arrive at a crossroads. One sees one's old conditioning as slavery and may then choose to abandon it in order to be free.

Shamans have always found wisdom in consulting animals to help them. The twelve animals of Liu Ho Pa Fa may be invoked to assist in the attainment of one's aspirations. Here is how they contribute:

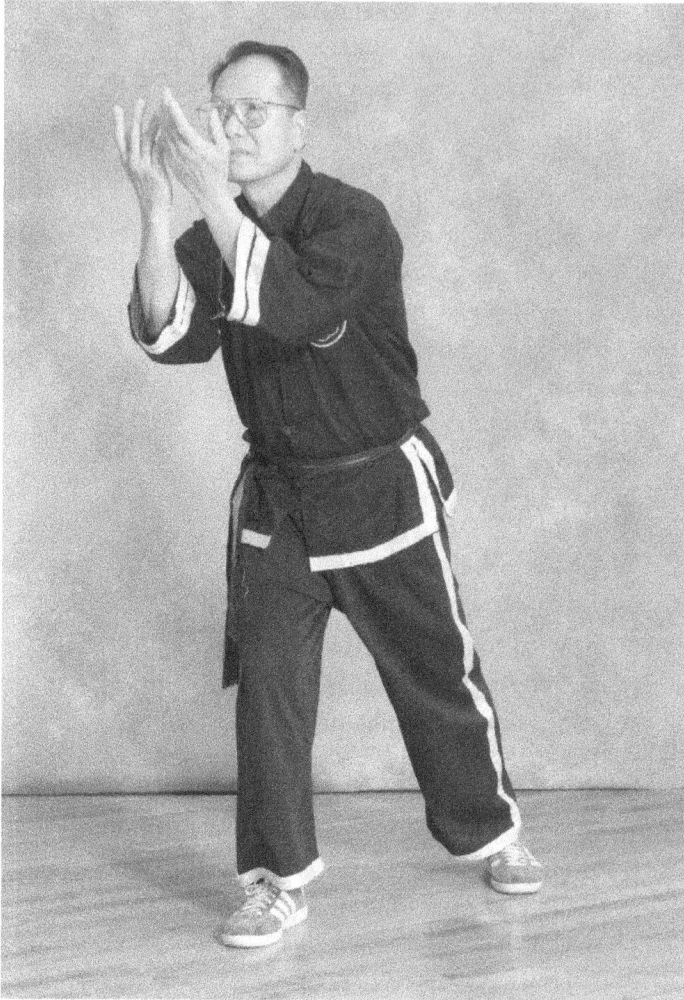

The **dragon** takes one's desire out of the limitations of the conditioned self, the ego, and brings it into the world of spirit.

The **lun** holds onto the desire until it is fulfilled.

The **pong** embraces all, then casts away the inessential so that the goal is reached.

The **mandarin** allows the will to proceed quickly while avoiding obstacles.

The **snake** makes one inaccessible to negativity.

The **ape** spirit takes only those inspirations that lead to progress and attainment, just as its physical counterpart swings from tree to tree on sturdy, secure vines.

The **bear** spirit dreams the dream of the heart and strikes down all opposition to its reification.

Grandmaster Wai-lun Choi demonstrates a movement of the Dragon posture from the Liu Ho Pa Fa 12 Animals set.

The **leopard** catches the most fleeting and elusive aspects of power.

The **crane** carries the aspiration to fulfillment.

The **goose** transforms energy so that the new adept may live in a new relationship with life.

The **eagle** lives in the heavens and swoops down to take from life only that which it desires.

The **tiger** is the full manifestation of the spirit: powerful, graceful, and invincible.

Sufi Master Hassan I Sabbah told his disciples that nothing is true, everything is permitted. Thus, one's root, one's center, one's dream has to do with personal choice. This is the important thing. The path one chooses is also personal, and if it is taken with intent and perseverance, it will take one where one wishes to go. At the core, one is either what one desires to be, or what others say that one is or should be.

It is my sincere hope that all will eventually choose joy and freedom. For Freyja, unto eternity, I aim my bow.

Psychology and T'ai-Chi

Ian Williamson, 2002

> Yang Cheng-Fu said that the quality of the mind should be as spacious and all-encompassing as the expanse of the universe.
> ~ *Wolfe Lowenthal in* **There are No Secrets**

If there is any quality of mind, anything psychological, that most especially belongs to T'ai-Chi, it is the quality of *sung*. This Chinese word is most commonly translated as "relaxation," but Western martial artists are astutely averse to simply leaving it there. Relax comes from Latin roots: re, meaning to go back, and lax, meaning looseness. To return to looseness, that is what is originally meant, and according to the Oxford English Dictionary, it has been associated with other positively connoted words throughout its history such as freedom and the release of tension.

But the fear that many martial artists have is that this word, relaxation, also indicates limpness and slackness, or ruan in Chinese. According to Cheng Man-Ch'ing, the beginner must first just focus on releasing tension, but eventually the practitioner must "contemplate the difference between going limp, which is lifeless, and the relaxation of a cat, which is completely vital and alert."

Or as Master T.T. Liang states, with his startling command of rhyme and rhythm in a second language, "Relax is not collapse." (He also used to say, incidentally, when our current masters Ray Hayward and Paul Abdella would pester him with questions, "These two masters come to bug me and mug me.") Tim Cartnell suggests images of pumping water or air through your open body. Essentially, looseness + vitality = *sung*.

We shouldn't forget either that relaxation also involves a return or a movement backward. It suggests other ideas prevalent in Taoism. For instance, Lao Tzu states, "Reversal is the movement of the Tao." Ai Yu Kuan writes in his preface to Sun Lu Tang's Xing *Yi Quan Xue*, "I was taught that what is born before one's body is born is called 'pre-natal,' and what is born after one's body is born is called 'post-natal'....The pre-natal Qi is the essence of Qi. It is peaceful and keeps the spirit in calmness."

Sun Lu Tang, in the same book, writes, "Sages can be versed in the way of inverse motion, can control the relation between Yin and Yang, manage the principle of creation, direct Liang Yi, grasp the key points, and go back to the pre-natal from the post-natal."

These points are remarkably similar to those found in Ruth Monroe's analysis of the birth trauma theory of Otto Rank, who was perhaps the least well known of Freud's prolific students. Monroe interprets Rank in the following way: "The person must regain a sense of unity with his world reminiscent of the intra-uterine state, but the unity cannot be effortlessly symbiotic. It must be based on a positive acceptance of the own will and the will of "others" at a new level of integration — indeed at constantly renewed levels of integration as the self expands and as "others" are selected or understood in an enlarging perspective. The progressive reintegration is accomplished mainly by love. The valid love relationship requires acceptance of the self-willing by another, and also acceptance of self-willing in another."

The psychological chain reactions spawned by these Eastern and Western psychological theories in themselves are relaxing and healthy because they rest upon an assumptive base: that people are naturally seeking a return to wholeness and unity symbolically expressed by the psychological state of the infant in the womb. This action is accomplished by a mature understanding of mutual love.

Nevertheless, this cannot be accomplished without constant, active, and creative reintegration of mind and body as we continue to recognize mental and physical patterns that are out of alignment and need attending and adjustment. Then we can feel this psychological state when we enter deeper states of meditation in T'ai-Chi, ever approximating more union and freedom of mind and movement.

One of the greatest qualities of T'ai-Chi is its obvious focus on creating greater union with our own bodies, which leads to a greater relaxation of our minds. As Lao-Tzu states, "The reason why I have great distress is that I have a body. If I had no body, what distress would I have?" By directing our effort at loosening our bodies, our bodies expand, or our minds expand to perceive them in more detail. Eventually in periods of enlightenment our minds and our selves even expand beyond our bodies to encompass greater horizons including other objects, people, and if you think as gigantically as Yang Cheng Fu, even the whole wide expanse of the universe.

A Pointed Question

Michael Pilla, 7th-Generation Lineageholder, 2002

Throughout the history of T'ai-Chi Ch'uan, T'ai-Chi's wisdom has been largely passed on by voice through legends, myths, and stories that are intended to convey technique and philosophy, and to inspire the search for truth and wisdom. Many of the stories told are epic and mythic in proportion. The story presented here is small, very human in scale, but hopefully of interest to the reader. It is a story of my sword and the expectations it can bring.

The sword and I have been together for many years. Through excellent teaching and hours of practice we have become skilled and expressive. As Master Liang once said, "The Solo Form is work, but the sword is play." Together, the sword and I play with our adversaries both real and imagined. We have become connected. Through this connection I have come to believe that each sword has a voice and spirit that we can learn to hear and learn from. Yes, the sword has become another teacher. To be blessed with adept teachers is indeed a great gift.

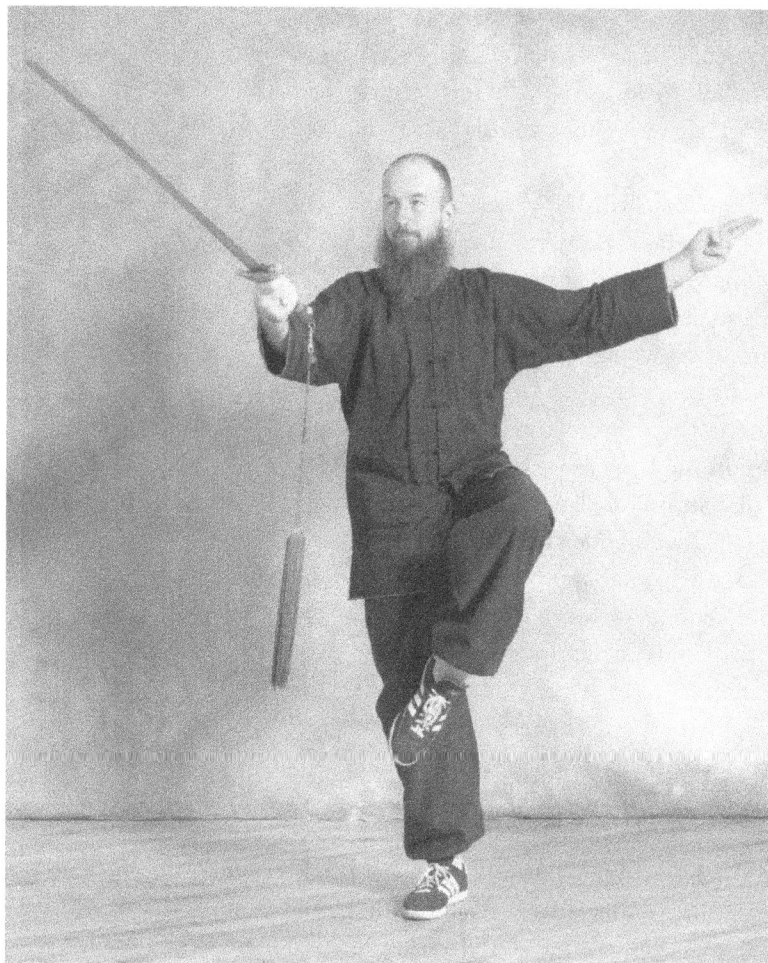

Ray Hayward demonstrates Send the Bird to the Top of the Bush posture for T'ai Chi sword with tassel.

So what does one do with a teacher that most consider inanimate? It speaks, but mainly to me. And when it teaches, I am most often the only one it shares its secrets with. It is a treasure, a secret between us.

Treasures are often hidden away for safekeeping, or proudly displayed for viewing. Neither seems appropriate for a true companion. A companion is someone who accompanies you. My sword most often travels with me in my truck. When I drive another vehicle I bring it along with me. And I prefer to drive long distances rather than fly just so that I can take the sword with me. Airport security frowns on sworded travelers.

Kids today are always fascinated when they see a sword. Certainly movies and television have brought an awareness that didn't exist when I was a kid. And my grandson has kept me informed about the level of interest kids have. Interest is one thing, but what about the meaning of having a sword? In other words, what does a child think when he encounters a sword, a weapon thing, in an everyday situation?

I'm a source of transport for my grandson, often taking him to and from school. I had recently taken to carrying the sword with me in the truck, when I came to school to take Jamin home. He saw me from the playground and knew that it was time to leave his friends behind and head for quieter times. He came to the door, opened it with a fling, tossed in his backpack, and then became suddenly cautious. I was confused. Before I could ask him what concerned him he said, "Grandpa, you have your sword with you." This was spoken with gravity and surprise.

I said, matter-of-factly, that I did have my sword with me. His concern only deepened. Then, as if he might be overheard by the wrong people, he said with concern and anticipation, "Are you expecting trouble?"

When I replied no, he asked, "Then why do you have it in the truck?" Before I had a chance to think I replied, "Because it's my friend and I feel better when my friend is with me." He nodded with a degree of understanding that was even greater than my own.

Now my grandson was also a fine teacher. It was only after the words had come out of my mouth that I realized the truth had been presented. Sometimes the best tool a good teacher has is a question. We only have to supply the answer.

THE RAGGED SWORD

Kim Husband, 7th-generation lineageholder, 2002

I have an old practice sword that used to belong to Master Liang. Ray gave it to me in the spring of 2001, I suspect because he grew tired of watching his advice on my form fall upon deaf ears and decided to turn me over to a higher authority. It's kind of a Big Deal to receive an item that used to belong to the Master, so I was a little disappointed by the lack of wonder the gift inspired — at first.

This sword is not a glamorous weapon, to say the least. Pretty much the opposite, really. It's just a single hunk of cast metal — no finely crafted blade fitted to a polished hilt and carved wooden grip. No slip-proof wrapping of cord on the smooth grip, either. No carefully weighted pommel to counterbalance the blade.

The blade itself is nicked and scratched and not even straight. It's certainly not sharp. The surface is a listless silver except for the grip, which my sweaty palm has tarnished to a dark grey, and it won't take a good shine no matter how hard I polish. The blade bears no etched dragons or Chinese characters, no blood groove or artisan's signature. The only ornamentation is a hole drilled in the pommel end for the attachment of a tassel. There's

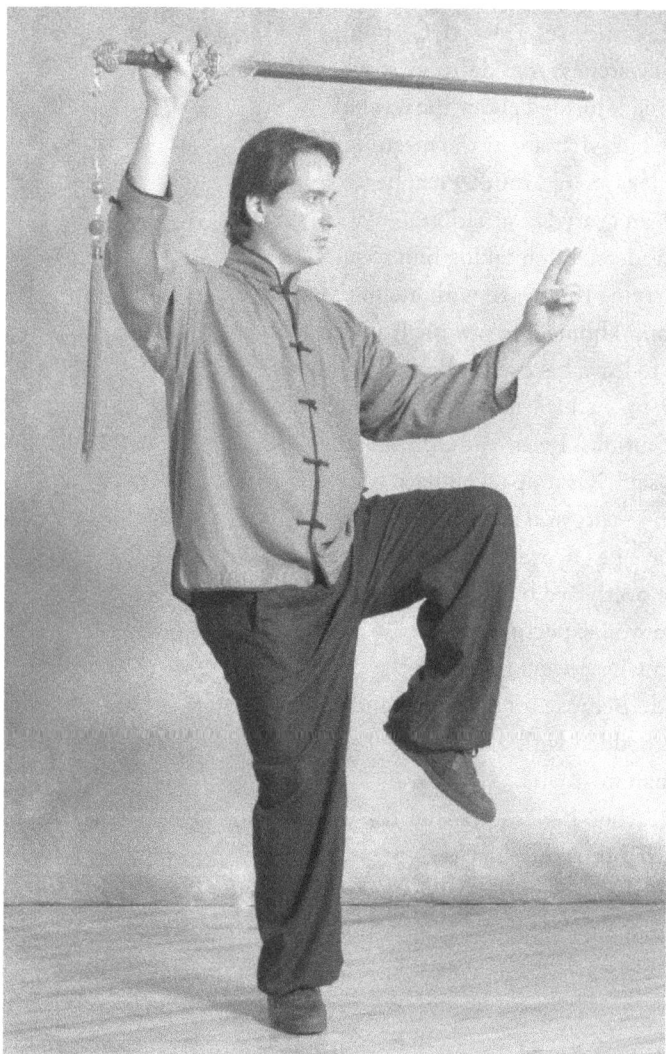

Paul Abdella demonstrates Chief Star of the Dipper for T'ai-Chi sword with tassel.

no scabbard, no painted or lacquered wooden home. No shiny brass fittings, no oiled sheath. The sword is kind of . . . ugly.

And yet, for an inanimate object, it's been a great teacher.

A line in the *Tao Te Ching* says "Those who speak do not know, and those who know do not speak." I begin to see what this means. With just a few words, Ray handed me this sword; with none at all it has told me things I didn't understand when I heard them spoken.

The blade's weight pulls me forward when I would hang back, slows me when I would rush. I must move it with my whole body; it won't listen to my puny hand alone. It doesn't distract my eye or my ego by being the prettiest weapon in the class. It does demand my full attention, or it will drag on the floor and take my balance with it. In short, it doesn't let me get away with much.

I'm still years away from doing the sword justice with my form, but that's OK. The important thing is that I'm paying attention and improving, albeit slowly.

The more important thing, though, is that I have the chance to do so. I have this chance because Master Liang chose to share his knowledge and his tools with his students, and they have chosen to share with me. Every student who has borrowed the ragged sword has learned from it. I promise I won't be the last.

Completing the Circle

Dianne Lefty, 7th-generation lineageholder, 2002

My first lesson in T'ai-Chi: I watched as the senior students appeared to glide across the floor with such grace and elegance, their movements fluid, each flowing slowly into the next. Everything coordinated — breathing, arms, legs, whole body, everything in motion. They seemed so peaceful and relaxed.

I went home and practiced over and over the few postures that I was shown, hoping to gain a glimmer of the feeling that the senior students were experiencing. My body felt awkward and clumsy as I moved from one posture to the next. Nothing was connected. I continued my practice several times a day, every day. I met with fellow students to practice and reinforce what I was learning.

Gradually, over time, it began — the feeling of fluidity in movement. I developed a library of T'ai-Chi books describing the postures, the philosophy and the T'ai-Chi Classics. I wanted to know, to understand, and to immerse myself totally in the study of T'ai-Chi. As my practice progressed, I thought of the great masters and the Classics and how everything was related in a circular unity. This art was so great, yes, it was perfect. The many years I had spent in formal education seemed lacking this great knowledge. How could this be?

I wanted to learn as much as possible. I studied the Solo Form, the weapons, Pa Kua, Hsing-I, the two-person form, push-hands, applications and Qigong, and am currently learning the Praying Mantis system. I believe they are interrelated and am hoping to integrate both systems in my T'ai-Chi studies.

So how does this amazing ancient Chinese art relate to my life? In so many ways, it would be impossible to identify and name them all. I find it especially helpful in stressful situations. I try to remain calm, relaxed, centered and rooted and to let the forceful energy flow past using the concepts of Ward Off and Roll Back, to name just a few. From my experience with the giant bird-eating spiders in the rain forest of Australia to my encounter with a grizzly bear on the trail in Denali, T'ai-Chi has helped me to survive.

When traveling to remote places in the world, I always try to find a "sacred" spot, a place that feels just right to practice the Solo Form. The energy is incredible.

When visiting China a few years ago, I went to the Temple of Heaven in Beijing to visit, but also to do T'ai-Chi in the park. I walked from group to group with my friend and translator until I found a group doing a form very similar to ours. My friend made the introductions and asked if it was all right for me to join them. The instructor was happy to have me, and after class invited me to study with him. At the conclusion of the practice, I presented the teacher with a gift from Ray. It was Master Liang's book. Even though the book was written in English, there was hope that someone would translate it into Chinese, and Master Liang's teachings would become part of the T'ai-Chi system in China. And so the circle is complete.

I thank Ray and Paul for their teaching and guidance, which allows me to participate in the knowledge they received directly from Master Liang.

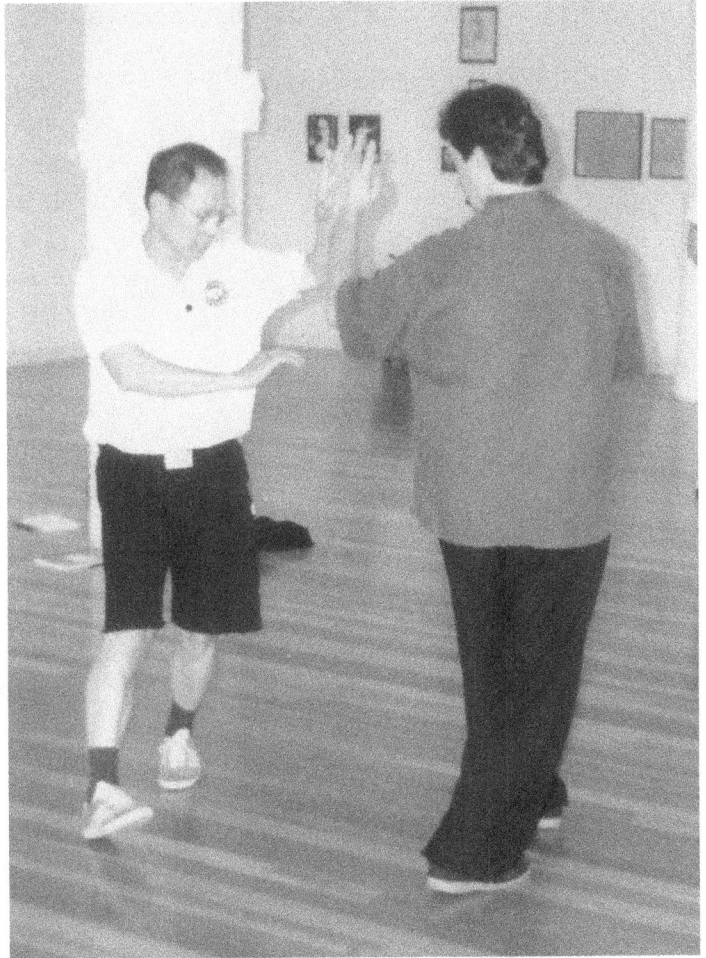

Grandmaster Choi and Paul Abdella practicing Pa Kua sensitivity.

What are the Rules?

Fred Sparks, 7th-generation lineageholder, 2003

I want to know what the rules are. I can't relax. It is not clear. Others seem to know, but no one will say. How do I act, what can I do, what should I avoid? Why don't they start on time?

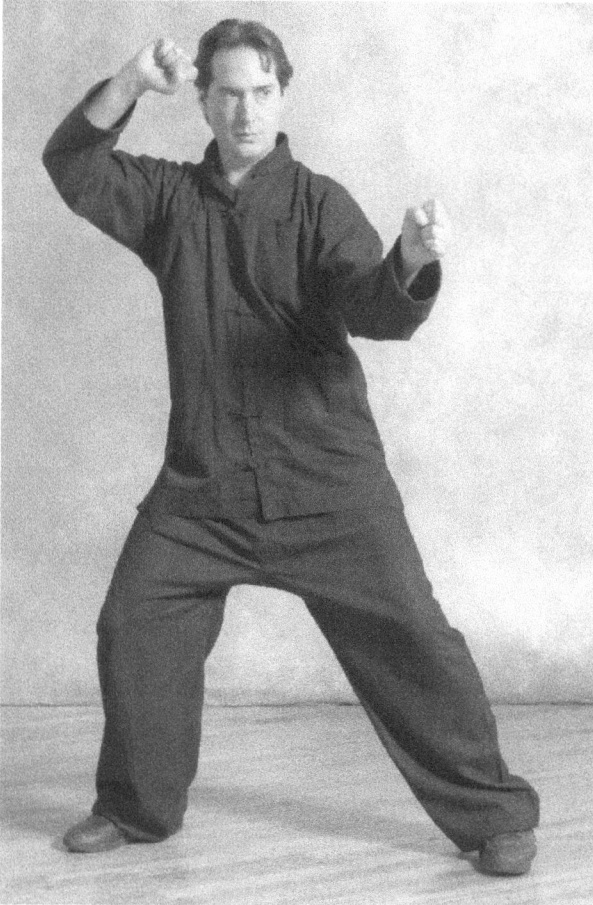

There is no start time, there is no conclusion, so you can relax. No one tells you, so you may relax. The rules are unwritten for you to relax. Yet we are human, and err, and worry. So I offer to you an invitation, unofficial, unapproved. If it helps you to relax, here are the rules I follow.

1. Respect our teachers.

They are there to give me something I want, I am there to absorb what I can. Listen. I may ask, but please don't question. The teacher tests me; the student does not test anyone. They are not perfect, they are not gurus, they are human. They can be so endearing that it is easy to forget my place and my manners. I will try what they give me before discarding. Whenever they offer a general, vague correction in class, I know that it is for me and that is for my benefit.

Paul Abdella demonstrates Bend the Bow to Shoot the Tiger.

2. Respect the teaching.

We all discover things along our paths. This information and practice is a culmination of many paths, passed on, and now placed at my feet. Will I take it and use it, or step on it? If I must voice disagreement, then I will disagree with myself, alone in the car, driving home.

3. Respect the school.

I will clean up after myself. Leave the property of the school, the teachers, and its students alone. When in doubt, I will ask permission.

4. Respect other students.

I will ask my partner's permission when pushing. I am willing to take no for an answer, and accept it without explanation. My classmates are free to participate or choose not to; I am not their judge. They have found a place where they feel comfortable, a place where they can relax and learn something. They feel safe here. So do I. Who am I to rob this from another person, and who is another to take this from me? As I choose to abide by this principle, I am infinitely free to relax and enjoy myself.

5. Relax.

I will leave the world at the door. Drop my burden. Breathe softly, slowly, smoothly. Feel the floor pushing against the bottoms of my feet...

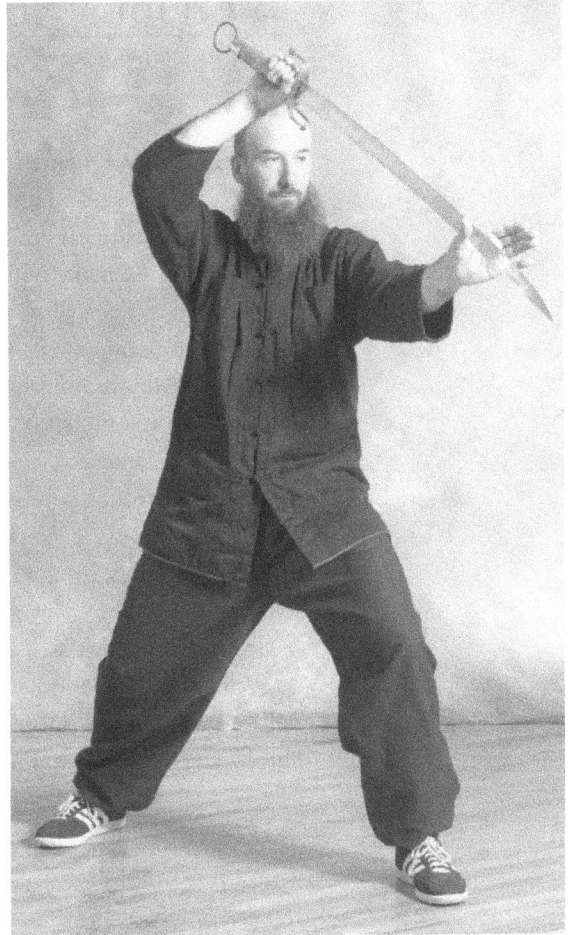

Ray Hayward demonstrates the Push the Knife Forward posture from the T'ai-Chi Sabre form.

So You Finished the Solo Form

Aaron Friday, 7th-generation lineageholder, 2002

Learning the sequence of the Solo Form is the first major undertaking of new T'ai-Chi students, and it really is quite an accomplishment. By the time your name appears in the newsletter under *Graduation News*, you've typically invested many hours imitating instructors, struggling with complex and difficult movements, and trying to memorize posture names that are at the same time poetic and bizarre ("Do what with the monkey?"). And for months you merely survived the form at the end of class, looking to others for clues about the next movement and feeling terribly conspicuous.

But now, through your own effort and persistence, you don't need help (well, not too much) to get through the form. You can do it on your own. As the saying goes, "Many have started — few have finished." You should be proud.

So what's the next step in your practice?

Well, your completion of the Solo Form entitles you to attend a multitude of more advanced classes that were previously off limits to you: The 2-Person San Shou, Pushing-Hands, Applications, and Weapons. If you have the interest, you are welcome and encouraged to attend these classes. They are important parts of the complete T'ai-Chi system, and each practice has its own purpose, challenges, and unique benefits. Plus, they are a lot of fun to learn.

Just keep two things in mind

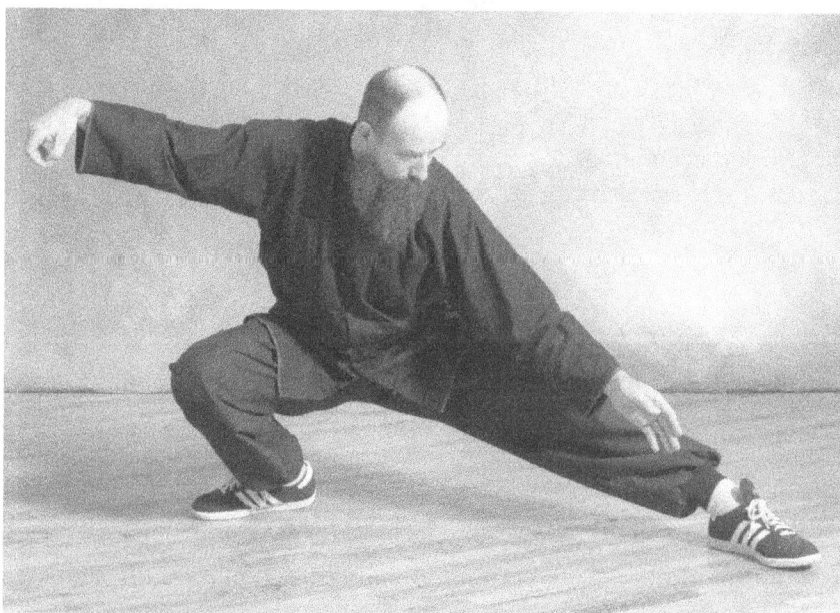

Ray Hayward demonstrates Squatting Single Whip.

before you join a new class: (1) it is always polite to ask the instructor if you can join the class, even if you've met the prerequisite, and (2) you still need to work on the Solo Form if you want to improve your T'ai-Chi.

The Solo Form is the foundation of all other T'ai-Chi practices that you will ever learn. Any improvements you make in your form will automatically benefit your understanding and execution of the Sword Form, Pushing Hands, and any other advanced practice you choose to pursue. It is the core exercise of your newly chosen art.

Traditionally, T'ai-Chi students are expected to adopt the Solo Form as a daily ritual. According to the masters:

Learners should practice regularly every morning or before going to bed. It is preferable to practice seven or eight times during the day-time; if one is hard pressed for time, then at least once in the morning and once in the evening.
  ~ *Yang Cheng-Fu*

...the daily exercise should be scheduled to have one round immediately after getting up, before the morning ablution; and the other immediately before going to bed for the night.
  ~ *Cheng Man-Ch'ing*

Practice in the morning, late afternoon, and in the evening. Go to bed, get up, and do it all over again. That is the way to succeed.
  ~ *T.T. Liang*

If you struggle with that kind of discipline, may I suggest that you just practice whenever you can, but try to do at least a little bit every day. To achieve and maintain a high level of health and well-being, we need quality exercise and stress relief on a daily basis. In addition, developing martial skill is a slow and painstaking process. Progress is hard to come by, and can easily be lost when we allow too much time to elapse between sessions. If you want the full benefits of T'ai-Chi, I believe you owe it to yourself to cultivate a daily Solo Form practice at home, in addition to what you're learning at the Studio. I can't think of a more worthwhile commitment to your own development.

To help you get started, I've listed some tips that I hope can guide or inspire you in your efforts. These are not my ideas, but ideas that I've either been given or have stolen from Paul, Ray, other teachers, and from books. I hope you can find something of value here.

Get out the Tape Measure. According to Masters Cheng Man-Ch'ing and T.T. Liang, three square feet is all the space you need to do the Solo Form. If you've seen the New Year's demonstration, you know that's the truth. Find a comfortable room in your home that provides enough space, rearrange the furniture to make more, or go outside if the weather is nice. If you are so inclined, a local park or gymnasium will work just as well.

Master the Jailhouse Step. The jailhouse step is a way of alternating forward and backward steps in the Solo Form so that you can practice in small spaces (like a jail cell) without bumping into things or disrupting the flow of the form. Students who practice in their homes are experts at this method of stepping.

Copy the Classes. If you're not sure what to work on, you can always copy the practice sequence used in the Solo Form classes. Start with some stretching and end with the whole form done smoothly. In between, you can practice meditation, hold postures, or work on a specific posture or section of the form. The most important thing, of course, is that you just do something.

Get the Tools. If you don't have these things yet, get them now. They will become essential learning aids for your home practice:

+ A notebook — Write down the theories, corrections, and practice methods you learn in class, as well as any insights you have. Refer to it when you practice at home, and you'll have no shortage of things to work on.

+ A metronome — Use it to control the tempo of your form, from very slow to very fast. You can try to use your own internal rhythm to go slower or faster, but it's not the same. A metronome is unforgiving, forcing you to control your own body and adapt to the tempo. Get one anywhere musical instruments are sold.

+ T'ai-Chi music on CD or audiocassette — Just push Play and start doing the form. Could it be any easier to practice? Buy it at the Studio.

- A timer — Use this when you've got a limited amount of time for practice. You could glance at the clock every minute or so, but this is very distracting. Better to just set a timer and get on with it. Buy one at Target or a similar store.

Measure In Hours. According to Sifu Choi, "It's not how long you've studied with a teacher, but how much you've practiced and how deeply you understand. We don't measure in years, we measure in hours and repetitions." There's the dreaded R-word. You'd think after all these generations, some brilliant master would have come up with a substitute for repetition, but so far no one has. Focus on the process, put in the hours, and do the reps. The benefits will follow.

Mix It Up. At the Studio, we are taught a multitude of different ways to practice the form: empty steps, holding the postures, holding the beats, different speeds/heights/frames, breath patterns, eyes closed, etc. These techniques help you develop proficiency in one or more aspects of the form. Use your personal practice time to explore them in more detail and keep your sessions interesting.

Do Your Homework. Have you ever received a correction to your form, and then three days later you couldn't remember what it was? This should not happen. Use your personal time to work through these corrections and assimilate them into your form. Repeat the movement over and over again until it feels natural, and you'll never forget it.

Follow the Correct Method. It is your instructor's job to impart the correct method to you. It is your job to learn it and make it your own through study, practice, and refinement. Whenever you practice the form at the Studio or at home, do your best to maintain the principles you have learned (e.g., relax, align with gravity, move smoothly, etc.). Calm down, be mindful of your movement, and be patient with yourself. Over time, you'll develop a keen sense of what is correct and what is not. Whenever you have questions, ask your teachers.

Be Introspective. Practicing at home is a time to analyze yourself and your form. Relax and get into your body. Feel your movements, and question everything. What is working for you? What isn't? Why do some postures feel natural and others do not? How can you let go of tension?

Try to answer these questions on your own first. If you get stuck or need guidance, ask your teachers the next time you are in class.

Do the Reading. Reading books and articles on T'ai-Chi can greatly improve your understanding and appreciation of the Solo Form. Learn as much as you can from reading, but start with this list. These materials were written specifically for you:

- *T'ai-Chi Ch'uan For Health and Self-Defense*, by Master T.T. Liang. This is our textbook of T'ai-Chi. According to Master Liang, 80% of his teachings are in this book. It's a priceless resource, but it cost me just $9.

- *T'ai-Chi Ch'uan: Lessons with Master T.T. Liang*, by Ray Hayward. Another priceless resource. These are transcriptions of Ray's own personal lessons with Master Liang, which he has generously made available to anyone with $20 and an interest in T'ai-Chi. Get this book from Ray directly.

- Articles in the newsletters and on the web site — These articles were written by Ray and Paul to offer further insights into what you're learning at the studio. They are available at no cost to you except for your time and attention. Visit http://www.tctaichi.com and read them.

And the final tip . . . **Persevere.** Practicing the form on a daily basis is a significant goal, one that is sure to challenge even the most confident and enthusiastic students when they actually try to do it. On certain days, most of us can muster the energy and enthusiasm to practice for several hours. But to practice every single day without fail, even for a few minutes, can prove to be much harder. Start slowly and be forgiving with yourself, but keep trying. At first, your small efforts might feel insignificant and even hopeless, but remember that all big accomplishments begin this way. With a small effort every day, your practice will soon become substantial, and you will be well on your way to receiving the full benefits of this magnificent form.

Good luck!

Clearing the Path

Kevin O'Grady, 7th-generation lineageholder, 2002

I came to the practice of T'ai-Chi eight years ago on the recommendation of a distant acquaintance. I had time on my hands, some curiosity, no experience, and few expectations. But within the matter of two hours I realized that I had stumbled upon something of profound personal importance. In part, it was the discovery of an activity that was relaxing, strengthening and invigorating. And in part, it was a discovery of something in me, something that was already there but obscured by the peripheral stuff and nonsense of life. My world began to become simpler and richer that day as T'ai-Chi served to clarify a path for me, not a goal, but a way of approaching life. It was a way that already existed within me, but that required some examination.

I choose the words "way" and "path" with deliberation, with reference to the philosophical Taoism of Lao Tzu and Chuang Tzu, to the *Book of Changes*, and to T. T. Liang's statements of the principles of T'ai-Chi. Time and again as I practice in the studio a line, phrase, or general concept from one or more of these sources will leap to mind, filling me with wonder at its simplicity and depth.

One of the more fundamental discoveries for me was the importance of change. I have grown up in the goal-oriented western world with its emphasis on static measures: data bits; sound bites; advertising images designed for consumption within a few seconds; poses and postures; degrees and belts; and the summation of an

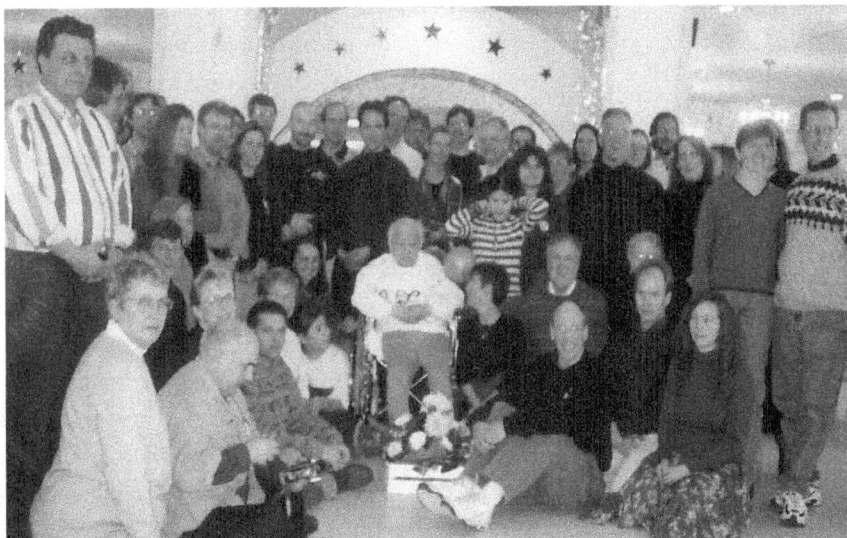

Master Liang's 100th bithday party, January 23rd, 2000.

entire life by focusing on where and how it ends. T'ai-Chi, in stark contrast, drew my attention to the importance of the path as distinct from the goal, to the movement between the points. For me the importance of the single-frame photo in the learning manual gave way to a need to understand the motions that came before and that will come after the photo (with the wholeness and connectedness of a string of pearls). To me, those changes are the heart of T'ai-Chi, and in my mind I have begun to rename some of the postures. Press becomes Pressing. Ward Off becomes Warding Off. Push becomes Pushing. "Posture," with its static connotation, is a word I have yet to discard. Perhaps "movement" is better.

With no particular goal to distract me the joy of repetition comes to the fore. If a movement feels clumsy, unbalanced, then I can repeat it and, since I had hoped to repeat it again and again, day in, day out, year in, year out, that repetition holds no negative import. I just do what I would do anyway. In this way, too, T'ai-Chi is relaxing, forgiving. To repeat a movement is the purpose of the practice. Here I think of Chapters 63 and 64 of the *Tao Te Ching* reminding me to pay attention to the small things, step by step.

Chapter 9 of the *Tao Te Ching* speaks of overfilling a bowl and of blunting the edge by over-sharpening the blade. As I proceed through a particular movement or movements I find rough spots, imbalances, that seem to persist, sometimes for many months. Typically, I will pay attention to the problem and throw myself into it, repetition after repetition after repetition, with seemingly no success. Then, frustrated, I cease to pay attention to the problem for a few days or weeks, only to find that when I again take up the practice my movement is as smooth as silk. It's tempting to think that if I can remove the imbalance by taking a week off, then I can become a master by ceasing to practice for years. But then I rein myself in with the reminder that it is the alternation between practice and rest, the change of pace, that allows me to untangle the knot.

The importance of two of the fundamental guidelines of T'ai-Chi, (1) relax and (2) sink, come to mind often in many aspects of daily life. I try to relax and sink into one leg while standing on ice as I slide into the driver's seat of my car. And there are many empty spots in the day where I can compose myself briefly by standing, relaxing and sinking: for a few moments in the elevator; in the airport waiting for a plane; and while waiting for access to the photocopier. Relaxing and sinking are also of benefit in more stressful situations: in disagreements with coworkers; in tests of will with one's children; and in navigating the freeway. While pushing a grocery cart in narrow, crowded, aisles I pay attention to my shoulders, unhooking them, relaxing, allowing them to sink. As they sink so, too, does my impatience.

The *Tao Te Ching* is rife with references to the distractions of the senses and to our overemphasis on learning, on knowledge, on analysis. Repetition of the movements helps to drive away distractions and analytical thought and to allow the mind and body to do nothing more than to be in motion. I've found that it is sometimes useful to reduce outward distractions by practicing the form blindfolded (closing my eyes is not sufficient as I will cheat when I feel uncomfortable). However, this tactic does more than simply remove distractions, it severs my orientation with much of the world outside of my body. My remaining senses focus on the feelings within my legs, the myriad tensions caused by efforts to counter minute, and sometimes major, imbalances. As such, it can be very exhausting. But, when I practice in this manner, I discover a tremendous sense of relaxation when I complete the Fair Ladies and move on to the non-stepping movements of Roll Back, Press, and Push. My relaxation increases even more when I remove the blindfold and practice with full vision. While practicing blindfolded it becomes clear to me that there is a line from my foot to my hip that is like a post, a post so strong and secure that it could carry my body weight several times over. When I find that post, rarely and briefly, my body feels weightless. The joy of such discovery far outweighs the embarrassment of losing my balance and stumbling into walls and pillars.

One of the more important principles of life which T'ai-Chi demonstrates to me is that of yielding, of retreating, of investing in loss, of meeting the hard with the soft, of discerning the substantial from the insubstantial. At its heart I take this principle to mean that it is of singular significance to pay attention to what is important and what is not. What is not important can be cast aside if necessary. What is important must be protected. And this distinction requires constant reassessment and it is this attentiveness, this awareness, that is one of the most rewarding aspects of life (whether it be joyful or otherwise).

I want to thank my distant acquaintance for pointing me to the Twin Cities T'ai-Chi Chuan studio eight years ago. There I met Ray and Paul. They gave me much more than a number of lessons in how to hold my arms and legs and how to tuck my bum under. They have helped enrich my life. I thank them.

Reflections of T'ai Chi Ch'uan

Diane Cannon, 7th-generation lineageholder, 2002

In the beginning....
> Learning to stand
> Learning to breathe
> Connecting my body, like a string of pearls.
> What is this feeling pouring into my hands?

Time goes on....
> Learning to swim
> Learning to be
> Counting the movements with each beat of the drum
> Where have you been all my life?

Hooked
> Learning to stand
> Learning to breathe
> Learning to swim
> Learning to be
> Warming my center as the music fills my bones
> Mind, body, spirit and breath, moving as one
> The commitment deepens
> The heart grows strong

Exploring unexpected paths
Knives, Swords, Spears and Fans enter my world
A Teacher, gentle and wise, retrieves a lost spirit
Brings her home
As the First Ray of Dawn lights the way

The Dance begins
> Refining, pushing, drilling
> Training mind and body
> Finding strength and power as the whole body moves
> One unit

Passion
       Never enough!
Respect
       Forevermore....

Life lessons at the foot of the Master
       Watching, listening, feeling overwhelmed as
       His two Disciples assist with loving eyes
       Tender walks, playful talks
       Feeding the soul with two plates
           Living the art of T'ai-Chi Ch'uan

A lifelong journey....
       Acknowledged
       Accepted
       Welcomed

Smiles, surprises, trials and celebrations
       T'ai-Chi Friends .... forever!
       With unending gratitude and respect to Sifu Ray Hayward,
           Diane Cannon

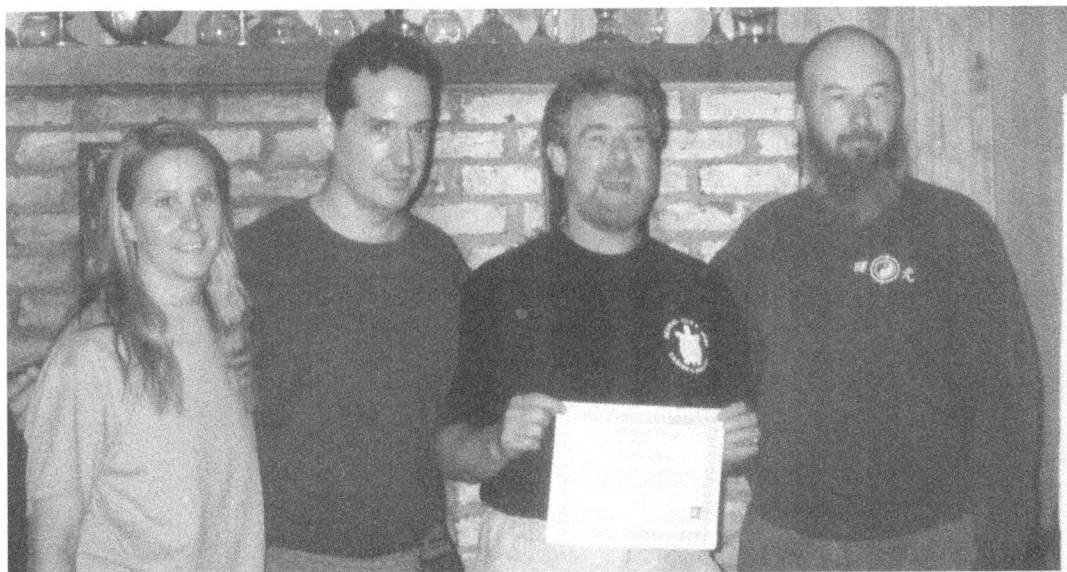

J. Richard Roy receives his disciple's certificate in 2000 from Ray Hayward and Paul Abdella. Disciple Diane Cannon is on the far left.

A True Master In Your Time

Diane Cannon, 7th-generation lineageholder, 2002

After one of many visits with Master Liang, Sifu Ray, Sifu Paul and many T'ai-Chi Friends, I felt completely overwhelmed by the love, respect and connections present. The experience was so powerful; it remained drumming in my mind and heart for a very long time. I embraced this "whole body memory" and can still easily return to that place and time, a true gift. Thank you to everyone that was present. I would like to share with you lyrics to a song I wrote that was inspired by that visit.

Lately, everywhere I go

A gently stroke upon my shoulder....
          Leads me back to you.
As we join our hands
I return to the source.

A dark corner, painting hours away
Brushing secrets — your masterpiece....
I raise the curtain to you sir
A freely giving man
Spreading wings of ancient Wisdom cross this land.

I wish I could have known you
          30 years or so ago...
When the sparkle in your sword would shine
          Tassels twirled so proud.
To witness all the beauty
          In your movement, soul and mind....
As unity reveals itself
A True Master in your time.

7 Stars Shooting through your eyes
Heavy hands still twist us down
Embrace the tiger in your heart...

Your spirit lives
       In one thousand friends —
Two chosen sons
With Gratitude
The waving hands of lightness
       Shine on you…

I wish I could have known you
       30 years or so ago…
When the sparkle in your sword would shine
       Tassels twirled so proud.
To witness all the beauty
       In your movement, soul and mind….
As unity reveals itself
A True Master in your time.

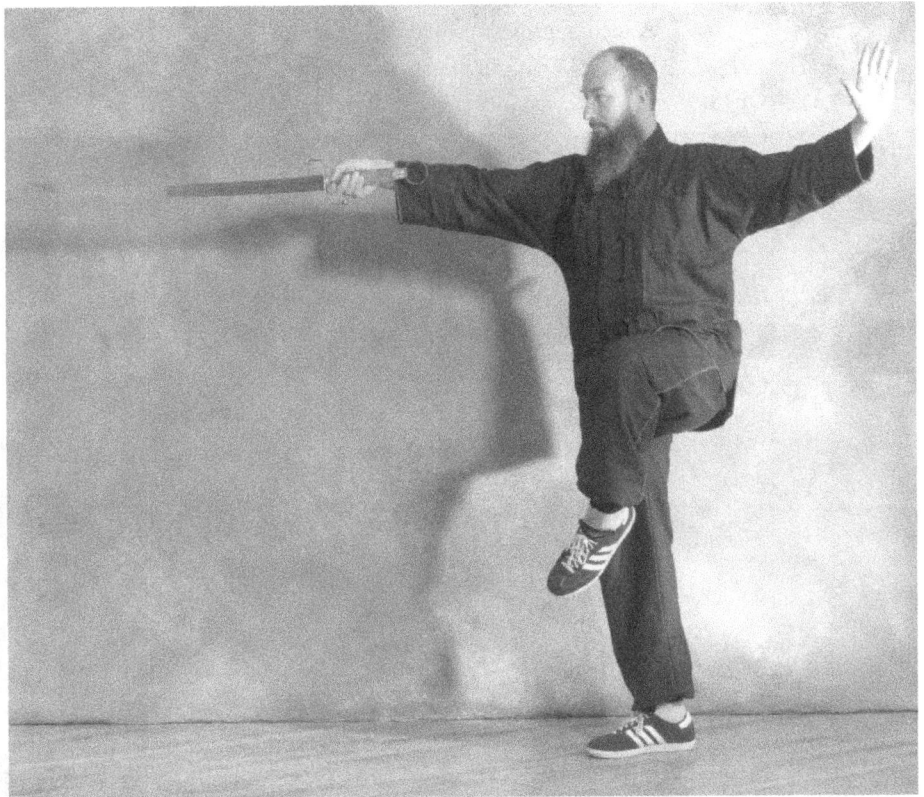

Ray Hayward demonstrating the Fair Lady Works at the Shuttle posture from the T'ai-Chi Sabre form.

A T'ai-Chi Experience

James Postiglione, 7th-generation lineageholder, 2003

A difficult task before me
To describe my T'ai-Chi experience
Something so important,
Such a part of me

Something started by chance,
Perhaps a hobby, no thought of more
Two teachers provide a taste
Then with Sifus Ray and Paul so much more

Through poor health and good
Practice, repetition and guidance
A feeling grows,
Subtlety changing flesh and spirit

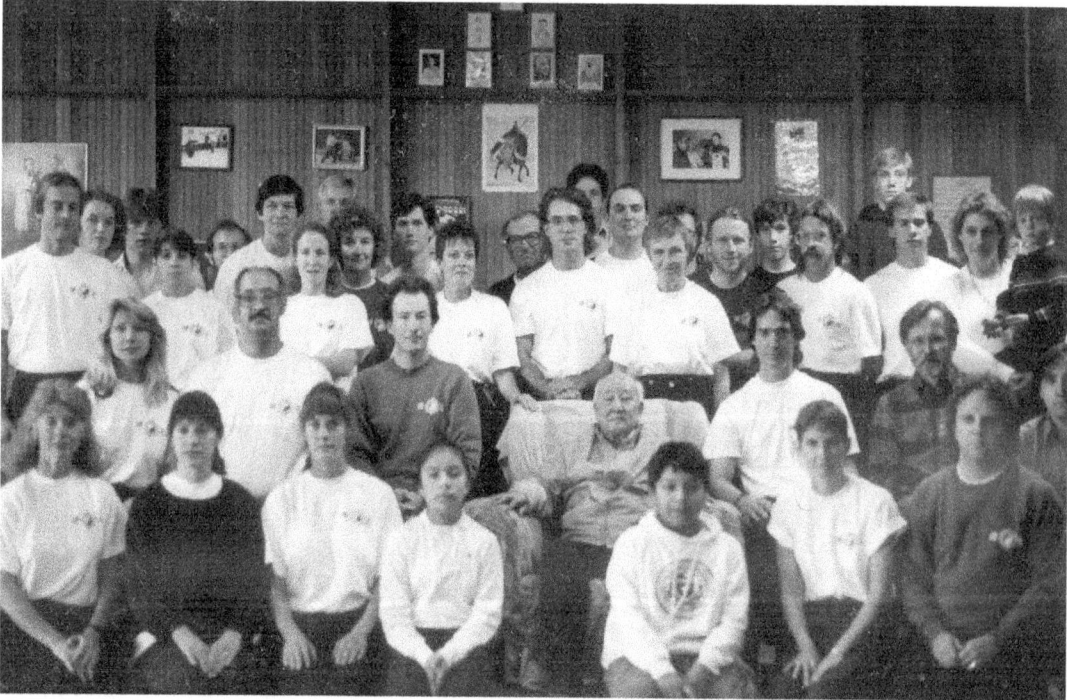

A farewell demonstration for Master T.T. Liang in St. Paul, Minnesota on October 23, 1988.

Bloodflow felt,
breath lowered,
legs strengthened,
sinews unraveled

Agitation ever present
aggressive reaction decreases
learn to wait, be still
a solution is found

Universal energy felt,
connection to heaven and earth once again
Collisions sensed, averted
Intensity diffused
Danger present,
Safety found

Progress is rapid, then slow
First small gains are measured in days
Months turn to years before whole body connected
Many levels hoped for some day

Time is precious, demands endless
Choices are many

T'ai-Chi brings great rewards
What value can there be on health?
On 20 minutes of peace?
On feeling inner chi?
On being centered and connected?
With practice rewards are many-fold.

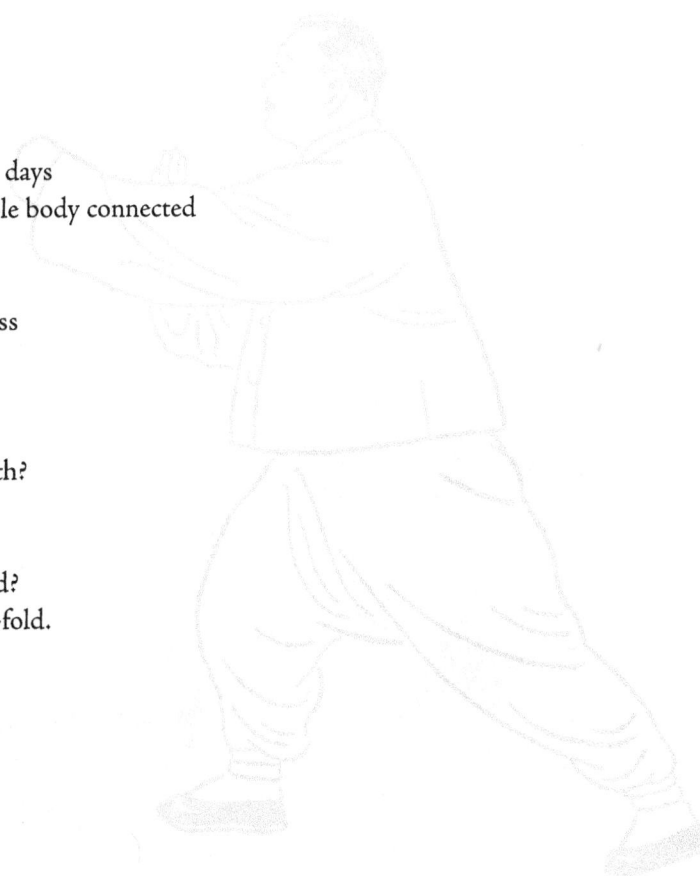

COUNTING POSTURES

TODD NESSER, 7TH-GENERATION LINEAGEHOLDER, 2002

One and two and three and —
     Sad, anxious, and angry
One and two and three and —
     Deadlines, errors, and expectations
One and two and three and —
     Exhaustion, tension, and headache
One and two and three —
     Loose, ease, and clear
One and two and three and —
     Relaxed, quiet and peaceful
One and two and three and —
     Revitalized, renewed, and happy

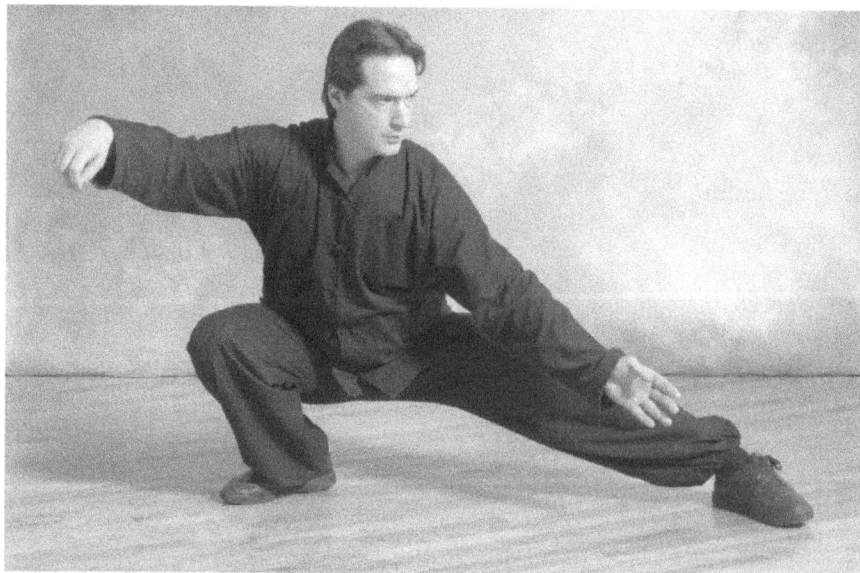

Paul Abdella demon-

FIELD OF CINNABAR

MORGAN GRAYCE WILLOW, 2002

In honor of Master T.T. Liang

His goal was to strengthen himself without interruption,
from desire, to intention, to first step — enticed
by this stream of the long river which rolls on.

Sick, reluctant to leave home and birth nation,
Liang heeded a fortuneteller's advice
in seeking to strengthen himself without interruption.

His liver poisoned by a life of dissipation,
he sought teachers of *T'ai-Chi*, began to practice
this stream of the long river which rolls on.

He learned to gather *ch'i*, to nurture its translation
through spine to all movements, without deficiency or excess.
In this way, he strengthened himself without interruption.

The teacher ready, now students appeared, asking him for instruction.
Retired, though not relieved from his calling, he passed
along his stream of that long river which rolls on.

Our practice honors his life-long celebration,
his goal now ours: To string pearls without severance or splice.
Having strengthened himself without interruption,
he continues. This stream, this long river rolls on.

Note: *Much of this largely found villanelle is drawn directly from Master T.T. Liang himself, from his book,* T'ai-Chi Ch'uan For Health and Self-Defense: Philosophy and Practice, *1977.*

A Ray of Silver

LaVonne Bunt, 2001

Ray,
In celebration of the culmination of your 25 years of T'ai-Chi mastery,
July 31, 2002. Congratulations!

An art is born in a quest for breath
a path of discovery is shaped by fluid movement caressing
the air, gently masking an issue of power from the center of a
mentor found

Practice and discipline are precursors of your journey
enduring respect kindled a route of passage with
Master Liang — teacher, mentor, friend
as a life quest toward mastery began

Ever studious, you ponder the essence of the spiritual quest
grounded in the resolve of a seeker on the path
you search the wisdom of sages condensing pearls
of those who have come before

As student now teacher your journey continues
each nuance taught echoes tempered refinements
of the mentor's lessons — as light, effortless movement
mirror the T'ai-Chi master, a mantle is being passed

Last Class

Elyse Duffy, 7th-generation lineageholder, 2003

Foreward

In the winter of 1994, Master T. T. Liang returned to Minnesota. Although at age 94 he was no longer teaching T'ai-Chi, he frequently observed classes on Monday nights. Those of us who were fortunate enough to be studying here at that time had the unique opportunity to experience the vastness of a great Master: the embodiment of yin and yang.

Monday, January 17, 1994

Another night at T'ai-Chi. It's been three weeks, and I guess I must like it. Anyway, I'm going four times a week.

There was a sign up tonight advertising a calligraphy class taught by Master T. T. Liang. He's the guy on the tattered green poster from Boston in the '70s. Ray and Paul's teacher. I've heard he's really famous, but what do I know?

I figure the class is on videotape, since it's only $5.00 and I think Liang still lives in Boston. Or maybe China. Anyway, why would some famous T'ai-Chi master come to Minnesota in January to teach calligraphy for $5.00 a class?

I think they should have put that on the sign. That it's a video class. So as not to be misleading.

I'm not really interested in a calligraphy class. What I really want is a Chinese Brush Painting class. But I figure this might be close. Besides, for $5.00, it's worth a try. Plus it should be fun to see a legendary master in action — even if it's just on videotape.

Monday, January 24, 1994

Got to the studio an hour earlier tonight for the calligraphy class. Confused, because the studio was open, no one there, and no video equipment. Then Ray showed up and said it was down the hall in Ruth Donhowe's studio. Ruth is in the Thursday day class and I thought it was awfully nice of her to contribute her studio for the video.

I wander around the corner, not sure which studio is Ruth's, but see an open door and peek inside. Paul is there, his back to me, fiddling with some paper and ink — getting ready for students.

I take a couple of steps inside, and see Paul isn't alone. Sitting next to him is this ancient-looking guy in scruffy, baggy sweats of indeterminate color. I stop in my tracks, momentarily stunned, while my brain readjusts its expectation: this is no videotape.

This is really the guy! Is it? T. T. Liang? Ninety-four-year-old T'ai-Chi Master?

Paul unrolls a bunch of parchment and the old man kinda grunts something at him. Paul calls him "Sir," and now I'm sure this really is *the* T. T. Liang. In the flesh. In Minnesota. In January?!?

I don't know if I should go on in or not. It's just Paul and Liang, and I don't know if there's a special protocol, or if I'm supposed to wait outside, or Oh, my God! He just spit!

I got out of there quick and ran to the bathroom to regroup. What in the hell was I getting into? For a minute, I thought I should just leave. I could just sneak out and come back in an hour. I don't think Paul saw me — I'm pretty sure he didn't — I never said I was taking the class — I'm sure there will be a bunch of other people in it — it's not like $5.00 will make or break this guy. The legendary T. T. Liang spit right on the floor!

Monday, February 21, 1994
I don't know what the hell I'm thinking. I'm still going to the calligraphy class, and I don't know why. Everyone else — there were only two others — have dropped out. Who can blame them?

Liang is one of the most cantankerous, irritating, irksome people I've ever met. I'd like to lock him in a room with my mother and see which one snaps first.

Tonight was more of the same. First the insults. Liang is obsessed with gender issues: he's constantly calling Paul a girl. Same thing with Ray when he watches classes. A constant barrage of "Are you a boy or a girl?" Paul and Ray just laugh it off, but I don't see any humor in it. It just makes me very uncomfortable.

Then there's the constant hawking and spitting. In the studio, Paul puts a wastebasket by his chair, and mostly he uses it. Once in a while he "misses," but I don't think it's an accident. He chortles every time he does it.

Monday, March 7, 1994

I don't think I can do this again. I feel bad, because if I quit going to class, it'll just be Liang and Paul, and I don't know, for some damn reason, I feel obligated to keep going. Obligated! I hate that.

It wouldn't be so bad if I were learning more. But Liang is impossible. After the requisite insults to Paul, he'll sometimes settle down and paint a character or two, and every so often, he'll actually say what the character is — its meaning.

Paul coaxes it out of him, but for every morsel he dishes out, there are two more insults. And several more gelatinous gobs of phlegm tossed into the wastebasket. I've gotten used to it enough that I hardly gag anymore.

He has a favorite passage that he copies over and over. It begins with the character for "man." Sometimes he'll recite more of it, Paul translating his faulty English.

When he's focused on the calligraphy, he works surprisingly quickly, and it's impossible (at least for me) to follow what he's doing. Every week, Paul patiently asks, "Master Liang, can you tell us which stroke comes first, second?" He's always rewarded with another barrage of "Are you girl? Why you have long hair? You girl. Pull down your pants. Let me see if you are girl or boy." Sometimes I just excuse myself and go to the bathroom for a respite.

Monday, March 21, 1994

Moth to a flame. That's what it feels like, and I ain't the flame. Liang is impossible and I find myself disliking him more every week. Yet I can't seem to quit. Something keeps drawing me to the calligraphy class, even though I dread the thought every Monday.

Tonight, in addition to the usual insults and spitting, he headed straight for the women's bathroom when Paul wasn't looking. He knows damn well which one is the men's. I ran and told Ray, because there was no way in hell I was going in there after him.

I've even tried convincing myself that his antics are Crazy Wisdom: like Gurdjieff's ditches and Rajneesh's "active" meditation; which I always thought was bullshit anyway — just a convenient excuse for a teacher to be abusive. And I think Liang's behavior is bullshit, too.

Then after class, Ray, Paul, Master Liang, and several students went to Baker's Square for dinner. I don't know why I went along, but I did. Liang's behavior doesn't improve much in public. I don't know what I was thinking, but I sure wasn't prepared for his eating habits. Suffice it to say that when he dumped his syrup-coated pancakes into his bowl of chicken noodle soup and delightedly chowed down, I nearly lost my dinner. Although, I must admit, the scene was so absurd, I almost laughed. Almost.

Monday, March 28, 1994

All week I was bothered by my continuing disdain for T. T. Liang. I've heard some amazing stories about him.

Like when he was arrested by the Japanese (he was a customs inspector in China during WWI). He was tortured. They broke his toes and feet. Paul says his feet are excruciating to look at — crumbled and broken and arthritic and deformed. I marvel, then, that he was ever able to walk again — let alone do T'ai-Chi. Of the half-dozen or so Chinese customs officers arrested and tortured, Liang was the only one to survive.

Or stories of his being a competitive ballroom dancer in the '40s! And that his love of dancing inspired his singular contribution to the Yang style long form: the addition of music.

I can't reconcile these stories with the cantankerous old man I see every Monday night and whose behavior continues to sicken and offend me. I dislike him intensely, and I hate myself for it.

I remember once hearing a story about Mother Therese. Someone asked her how she could tolerate the physical putrefaction of the lepers she cared for: how could she stand the smell of their rotting bodies, the sight of their festering wounds. She replied, that when one serves, one rises above and notices none of these things. I wonder if there is a way I can serve Liang. Something that will take me beyond my anger, my distaste, my judgments.

Driving to the studio, I suddenly stop at Trotter's bakery, not sure why. Inside, I pick out a couple of their oversized cupcakes: chocolate, chocolate chip and turtle. I ask for them in a box, grab a handful of extra napkins, and head for the studio.

Monday, April 11, 1994

I'm now the "cake lady." Liang loves the boxes of sweets I bring every Monday now, and even though I've brought cookies, scones, cup cakes, and bear claws, they're all just cakes to him, and I'm the cake lady.

The calligraphy class is easier now. For whatever reason, Liang's insults don't bother me so much anymore, and there seem to be fewer of them. His focus is more on the calligraphy, and tonight the most amazing thing happened. Halfway through class, he became very quiet and still.

Time seemed to slow and I watched as his arthritic, 94-year-old fingers picked up the brush and held it with the delicacy of a lover. And from this beloved issued a softness, a suppleness, a beauty that defied the crippled hands that yielded it — or to it.

I hold my breath (T'ai-Chi principles be damned), afraid to break the spell.

The characters flow from the brush one after another: delicate foot soldiers marching down the page from top to bottom. They remind me of those hundreds of ancient Chinese soldiers they excavated from a grave. Except Liang's characters are more delicate, ephemeral and speak not of war, but of peace — the peace of the soul.

As suddenly as he began, he is done. Quietly, Paul asks — for perhaps the hundredth time — if he will show the order of strokes in each of the characters.

His response is to spit. This time he misses the waste basket, my stomach turns, and I excuse myself to use the bathroom.

Monday, April 25, 1994

My hand is shaking. I don't know if I can write all of this, but I want to try.

Liang was unusually irksome tonight, and despite my softening heart, I felt myself losing patience. Then, ten or fifteen minutes before class ended, Paul excused himself and said he had to deal with something. He'd be back shortly.

I couldn't believe he was leaving me alone with Liang! I'd never been alone with him before. How would I handle him if he just decided to get up and head down the stairs? Or to the women's bathroom? Or what if he started asking me to drop my pants so he could see if I was a boy or a girl?

I would have panicked, except Paul was already gone, and panicking didn't seem like the most auspicious thing to do, alone in a room with Liang. So I turned back to him, smiling, but shaking inside, terrified of what he would say or do.

The next few minutes passed without incident, and I just kept copying out the characters from his favorite piece as best I could. Then he grunted at me and I steeled myself for the worst. But all he wanted was a clean sheet of paper, and I could do that easily enough.

I stopped my copying to see what he would do next. It was his favorite piece, the one I'd seen him write a dozen times before. But he'd gone into that quiet place again, where he turned to the calligraphy with focused, centered mind, and his wizened, crippled fingers became light and delicate, like the petals of a rare orchid, floating on the wind. And from them flowed the most elegant, graceful, perfected characters. I didn't care what they meant. I didn't care that he was insulting, and bad-mannered and cantankerous. I only cared that the ink flowed from his brush like a weightless dance — as light and graceful as any ballerina flowing into a liquid arabesque.

When he finished, I let out my breath, and said it was time to clean up. But Master Liang demanded a pencil, and I handed it to him, having no idea what he wanted with it.

Then, in amazement, I watched as he numbered every single stroke of every single character in the entire piece. Sometimes he would count aloud: *one! two! three! four!* sounding just like he did on the music tape.

When he was done, he thrust the paper into my hand with the words: *Now practice!*

I thanked him, at least I think I thanked him. I certainly meant to. But I was so flabbergasted, I'm not sure that I had a voice. I was frozen to the spot, and only jarred from my stupor when I realized Liang was headed, unescorted, out the door. Luckily Paul had just returned and herded him back inside.

There is no more time for astonishment. I help Paul clean up. He and Master Liang leave and I'm left holding the calligraphy. A tear drops onto the page and I wipe it quickly away, lest it mar this treasure.

Afterword

The next week, there was no calligraphy class. Paul told me that Master Liang refused to change out of his pajamas. So, while it was May, it was still too cold to go out in PJs and rather than change, Master Liang decided to stay home.

While he did return — for more than a year — to observe Monday night classes, and to continue his relentless assault on Ray and Paul's gender identities, the calligraphy class on April 25, 1994 was the last class T. T. Liang taught at the Twin Cities T'ai-Chi Ch'uan studio.

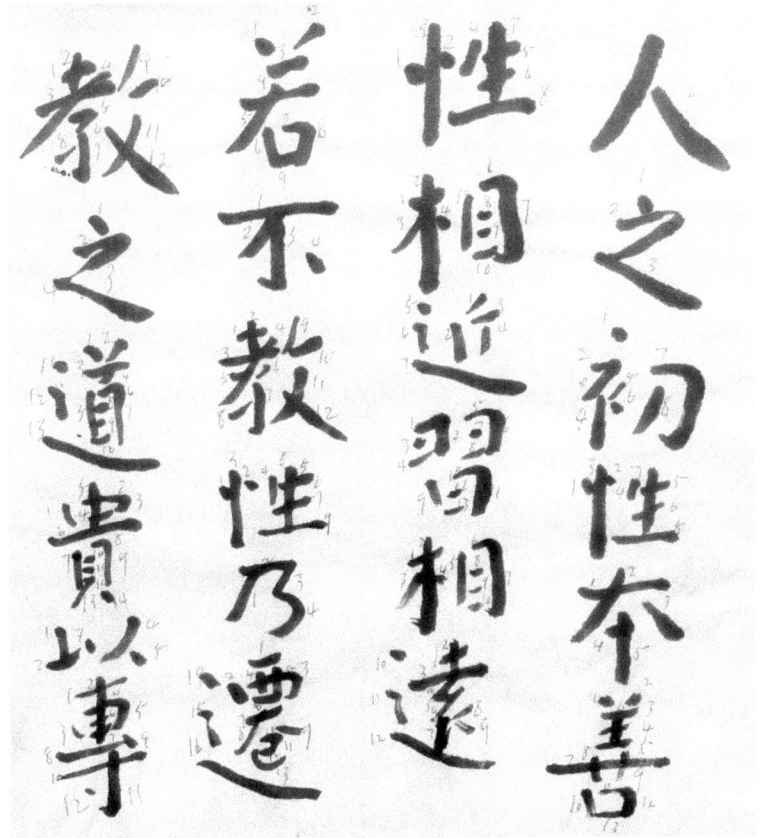

人之初性本善
性相近習相遠
若不教性乃遷
教之道貴以專

Master Liang's calligraphy (with numbered strokes) from his last class.

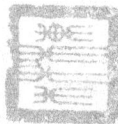

The disciple certificate written in Chinese by Master T.T. Liang for Ray Hayward (Shu-kuang) and Paul Abdella (Huei-ming) on November 11th, 1988 in St. Cloud, Minnesota.

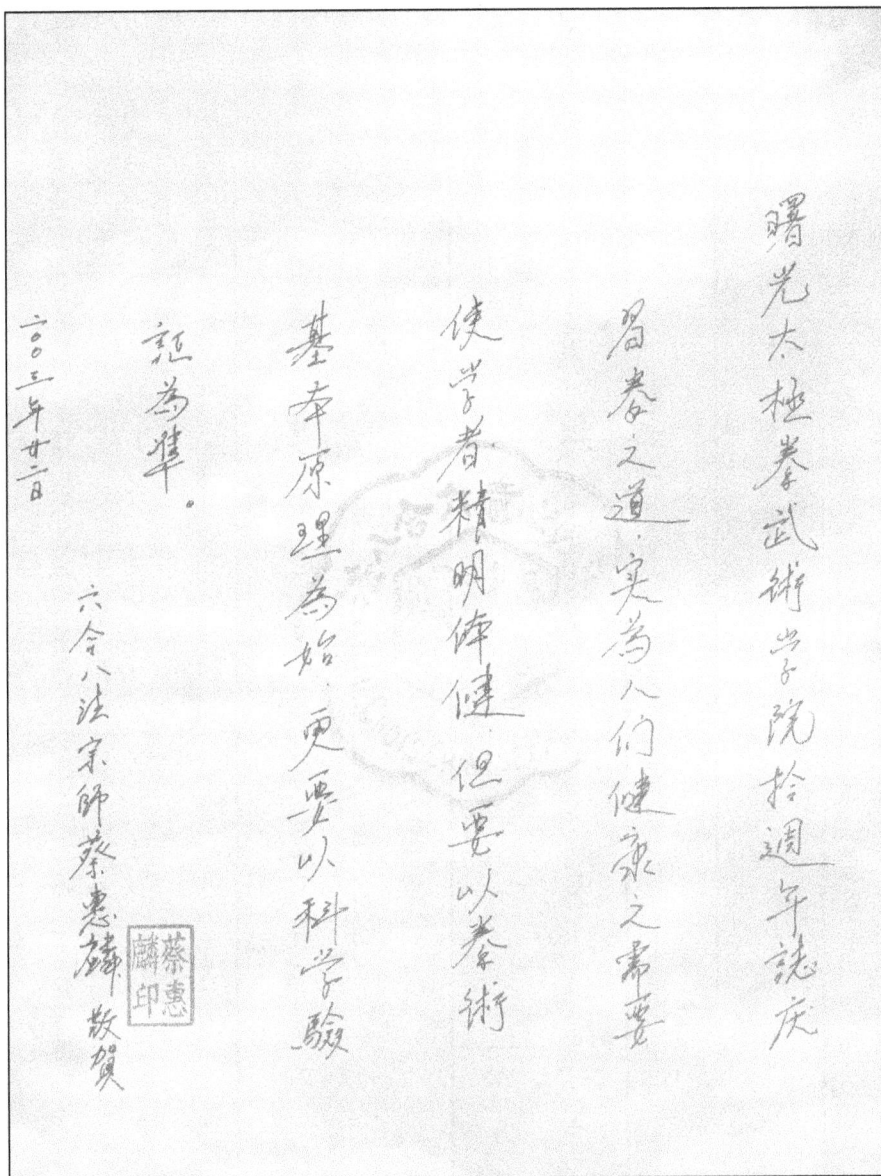

曙光太極拳武術學院拾週年誌慶

習拳之道，實為人們健康之需要

使學者精明體健，但要以拳術

基本原理為始，更要以科學驗

証為準。

六合八法宗師蔡惠麟 敬賀

二〇〇三年廿二日

Grandmaster Wai-lun Choi presented this calligraphy to Twin Cities T'ai-Chi Ch'uan for the Studio's 10th anniversary demonstration. The calligraphy reads, "For Shu-kuang's Twin Cities T'ai-Chi Ch'uan Studio's 10 year anniversary. To learn Martial Arts is the deepest way for people to improve their health, develop their minds, and make their body strong. One must understand and apply the basic principles and use science as a standard to prove their correctness.

With respect and congratulations
Liu Ho Pa Fa Grandmaster Wai-lun Choi
February 22, 2003

Twin Cities T'ai-chi Ch'uan Studio's
Yang-Style Lineage

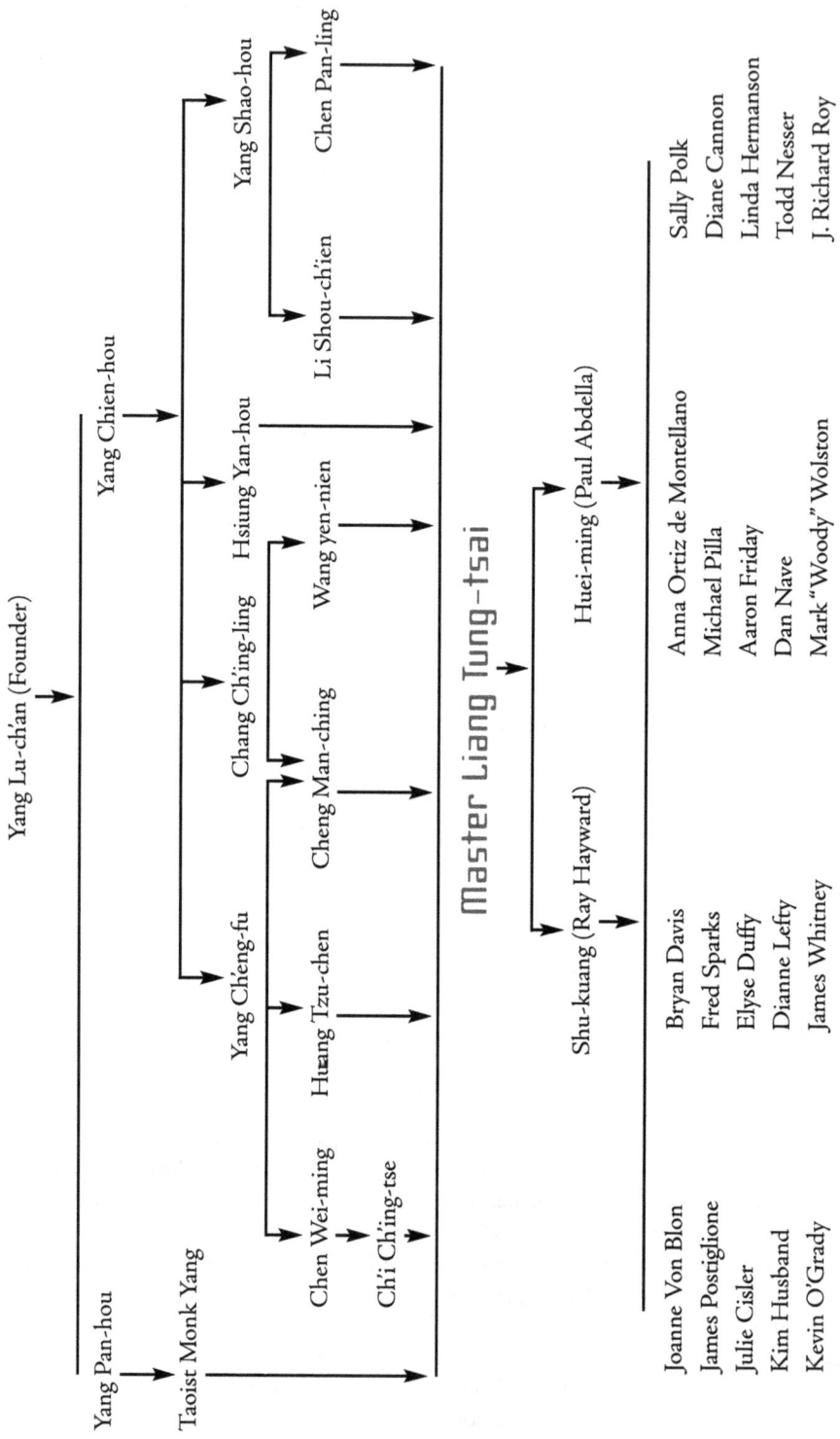

Yang Lu-ch'an (Founder)

Yang Pan-hou

Yang Chien-hou

Taoist Monk Yang

Yang Ch'eng-fu

Chang Ch'ing-ling

Hsiung Yan-hou

Yang Shao-hou

Chen Wei-ming

Huang Tzu-chen

Cheng Man-ching

Wang yen-nien

Li Shou-ch'ien

Chen Pan-ling

Ch'i Ch'ing-tse

Master Liang Tung-tsai

Shu-kuang (Ray Hayward)

Huei-ming (Paul Abdella)

Joanne Von Blon
James Postiglione
Julie Cisler
Kim Husband
Kevin O'Grady

Bryan Davis
Fred Sparks
Elyse Duffy
Dianne Lefty
James Whitney

Anna Ortiz de Montellano
Michael Pilla
Aaron Friday
Dan Nave
Mark "Woody" Wolston

Sally Polk
Diane Cannon
Linda Hermanson
Todd Nesser
J. Richard Roy

Index

About the Author

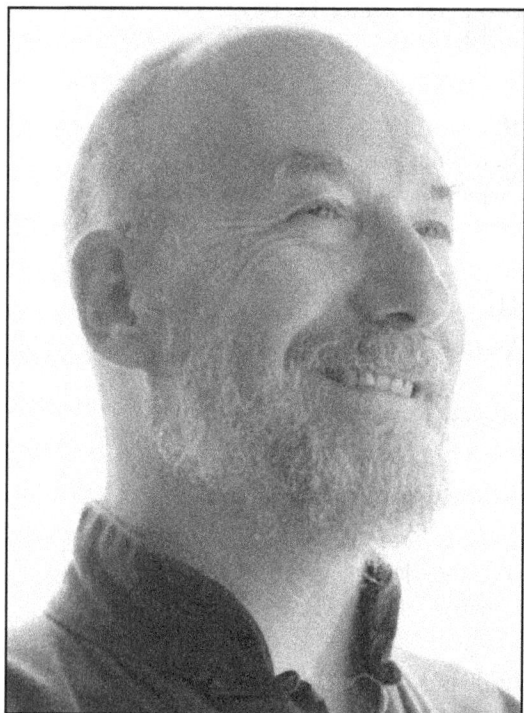

Sifu Ray Hayward (Shu-Kuang) began his health maintenance and Martial Arts training in 1973, studying Kenpo Karate and Jiu-Jitsu. In 1977, he met and began study with Master T.T. Liang in Boston. Ray learned the complete Yang Style T'ai-Chi Ch'uan system from Master Liang, as well as Praying Mantis, Ch'i-Kung, Taoist Meditation, Ch'in-Na, Wu Dang Sword and various weapons. In 1984, Ray moved to Minnesota to continue studying with Master Liang. In 1988, Sifu Hayward passed through a formal ceremony to become an inner-door disciple of Master T.T. Liang.

Ray studied Northern Shao-Lin Long Fist, Praying Mantis, Pa-Kua Chang, Hsing-Yi Ch'uan, Chen Style T'ai-Chi Ch'uan, Ch'in-Na, and various weapons with Dr. Leung Kay-chi. He studied Northern 7-Star Praying Mantis and Fanzi Eagle Claw with the late Sifu Lo Man-biu.

Ray learned Taoist Meditation, Qigong, 5 Animal Frolics, and T'ai-Chi Ruler from Masters Paul B. Gallagher and Kenneth S. Cohen.

Other teachers include Master William C.C. Chen, Master B.P. Chan, Mr. Heinz Rottmann, Mr. Li Wang, and Sensei John Duncan.

Sifu Hayward rounded out his martial arts education by studying with Liu Ho Ba Fa Grandmaster Wai-lun Choi, learning Hsing-Yi Ch'uan, Pa-Kua Chang, Y'i-Ch'uan, Qigong, Taoist Meditation, and Wu Dang Sword.

Ray privately studied Kwong Sai Jook Lum Southern Praying Mantis, Sin-Kung and Calligraphy with Grandmaster Gin-foon Mark.

Ray currently studies Luk Hop Bat Fat with Grandmaster Wai-Lun Choi, and Modern Tactical Martial Arts with Master Rob Jones. He studies the breath technique and methods of Wim Hof and Stig Severinsen.

With a deep interest in spirituality and meditation, Ray has explored many Eastern religions, focusing on Taoism and Sufism. Ray studied 11 years with Sufi Master, Shaykh Nazim al Haqqanni an Naqshbandi. He has also studied Hypnotherapy, Psychology, and is certified in the Healing

Tao System. He has made extensive research and study concerning the Western Mysteries, including Alchemy, Freemasonry, the Knights Templar, Rune Lore, the Rosicrucians, Druidry, Celtic history, and Rosslyn Chapel, studying with such masters as David Sinclair Bouschor, Joseph Lang, Charles W. Nelson, Timothy W. Hogan, and Philip & Stephanie Carr-Gomm. In 2010, Ray became a Druid Graduate in the Order of Bards, Ovates and Druids.

In 1979, Ray began teaching T'ai-Chi as an assistant under Master T.T. Liang in Boston, and then as a full-time instructor in Minnesota from 1984 to the present. From 1984 to 2016, he was the chief instructor for the Twin Cities T'ai-Chi Ch'uan Studio. He currently runs his own school, Mindful Motion Tai-Chi Academy, in Minneapolis. Ray has taught T'ai-Chi at the Sister Kenny Pain Clinic at Abbott Northwestern Hospital, Hazelden Treatment Center, Courage Center, General Mills World Headquarters, Virginia Piper Cancer Center, Minneapolis Public Schools, the Northfield Community Education Department, and Carelton College P.E. and Rec Department. He has also conducted seminars, workshops, and retreats throughout the United States. Internationally, Ray has taught in Winnipeg, Canada, and in London, England.

Sifu Ray Hayward has taught martial arts to hundreds of people, particularly T'ai-Chi Ch'uan, as a way to gain health, peace of mind, physical confidence, and a state of well-being. His goal is to empower, not overpower, others.

"Forty years is a short time when exploring the mysteries and experiencing the benefits of the art of T'ai-Chi Ch'uan."

-Ray Hayward

Contact Information

Mindful Motion Tai-Chi Academy
www.mindfulmotiontaichi.com
Facebook: facebook.com/Mindful-Motion-Tai-Chi-Academy

Ray Hayward Enterprises
www.rayhayward.com
skrayhayward@gmail.com

Grandmaster Wai-lun Choi
www.liuhopafa.com

Paul Gallagher
www.totaltaichi.com

Kenneth Cohen
www.qigonghealing.com

Gin-foon Mark
www.masterginfoonmark.com

Dr. Leung Kay-Chi
www.jiannshyongkungfu.com

Order of Bards, Ovates and Druids
www.druidry.org

Timothy W. Hogan
www.lulu.com/spotlight/Emerys

Sensei Rob Jones
rrpj72@gmail.com

Julie Cisler (graphic design & production)
juliecisler13@hotmail.com

www.ingramcontent.com/pod-product-compliance
Lightning Source LLC
Chambersburg PA
CBHW080331270326
41927CB00014B/3182